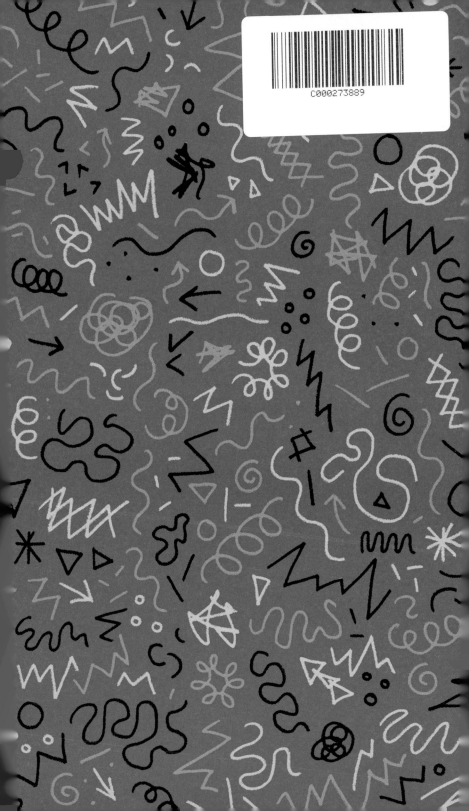

C000273889

SCATTER BRAIN

HOW I FINALLY GOT OFF
THE **ADHD** ROLLERCOASTER
AND BECAME THE OWNER OF A VERY TIDY SOCK DRAWER

SHAPARAK KHORSANDI

Vermilion

For my mum, Fatemeh Khorsandi

1

Vermilion, an imprint of Ebury Publishing
20 Vauxhall Bridge Road
London SW1V 2SA

Vermilion is part of the Penguin Random House group of companies
whose addresses can be found at global.penguinrandomhouse.com

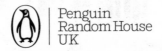

Penguin
Random House
UK

First published by Vermilion in 2023

www.penguin.co.uk

A CIP catalogue record for this book is available from the British Library

ISBN 9781785044199

Printed and bound in Great Britain by Clays Ltd, Elcograf S.p.A.

The authorised representative in the EEA is Penguin Random House
Ireland, Morrison Chambers, 32 Nassau Street, Dublin D02 YH68.

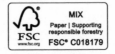

Penguin Random House is committed to a sustainable future
for our business, our readers and our planet. This book is
made from Forest Stewardship Council® certified paper.

CONTENTS

CHAPTER ONE

'In my twenty-three years as a psychotherapist, I've seen the same patterns appearing. Those of us with ADHD, who struggled at school, will immediately recognise the torment and anguish hidden beneath a defensive layer of humour. That sort of classroom and playground trauma leaves indelible marks.

ADHD is not simply about diagnosis, it's often about the trauma one endures as a young person as a result of undiagnosed ADHD.'

Ian King-Brown, Psychoanalytical Psychotherapist

I am lying: this is not chapter one. It's the introduction. Why am I tricking you into reading it? Well, because if you are anything like me you might skip the intro. I have ADHD (Attention Deficit Hyperactivity Disorder) and INTRODUC-TION at the top of the page in a book feels to me like the warm-up act that comes on at a gig, before the lights have fully dimmed and there's still time to grab a beer or go to the loo. *Just tell me the stuff!* I think. 'Go straight to the main bit! Just gimme the facts, tell me the story, NOW!' I mutter to myself. 'I don't need it to do a little dance for me before it starts.'

This bit *is* important, though, so please read to the end. If you have ADHD too, slap yourself, do a twirl, sing, 'I've got a Loverly Bunch of Coconuts' – whatever you have to do to stay focused.

All my life, people had given me the nickname 'Scatty Shappi', and I never contested it. There was, after all, endless proof. I was always losing things, getting times wrong and being unsure of where I was meant to be or what I was meant to be doing. I was madly impulsive; rarely thought things through. I could not start things, I certainly couldn't finish anything, yet loaded my plate with tasks and activities: 'Yes, I'll do that! I will be there! Dorset and Mull of Kintyre in the same day? Sure! No problem!' I lived in a fog of daydreams. I was socially quite clueless, insanely sensitive and had a real problem with sitting still and concentrating. And by 'real problem', I mean I could not do it. I had a temper, too. Not an ordinary temper but a tired-hungry-two-year-old-who's-broken-her-banana temper, which is scary on a grown woman.

Finally, in my mid-forties, during the Covid-19 lockdown, I was diagnosed with Attention Deficit Hyperactivity Disorder (ADHD). I learned that my brain has chemical deficiencies which affect my executive functions.

I started on the road to getting support and beginning to understand how my brain works. It all started with an absolute meltdown over a box of chocolates.

It was lockdown, there was a lot of uncertainty, and when my children squabbled a little over how best to open the box of Milk Tray I hurled it across the room, burst into tears and ran out of the house with no shoes on.

My reaction was born from my ADHD affecting my ability to process emotions and react in emotionally appropriate ways. If you notice a box of chocolates has a bomb attached to it and it's ticking, then you can justify hurling it away while screaming. If your children have a *mild* disagreement about how best to open said box of chocolates, it's trickier to justify this reaction.

Frequent over-the-top reactions affected not just me, but the people I love, and occasionally people on the bus who played their music out loud. At other times, I became a compliant people-pleaser to the rest of the world in order to mask my ADHD. I had, unconsciously, throughout my life, become dependent on harmful ways to mask and self-medicate for my ADHD. Compulsive eating, bulimia, binge-drinking and other obsessive-compulsive behaviours had dogged me throughout adulthood.

I began to read about ADHD. Friends I made while walking my dog in the park told me they knew people who had ADHD and recommended an online magazine to read (it's called *ADDitude*) and podcasts to listen to. This allowed me to start to make sense of myself. I felt like how I imagine Tarzan did when he realised the apes were not his blood family, that he was really a human, so it was okay that eating maggots and having sex with chimpanzees wasn't for him. What a relief!

I found a therapist who specialised in ADHD. I had never had holistic therapy before, where I didn't feel like I was a problem to 'fix', but a person who needed support. My therapist helped me find the words to express the decades of frustration, and he was empathetic to all of it. I also saw a psychiatrist who diagnosed me with the condition, and for the last year or two I have been learning about ADHD, how it affects me, and I have also started coming to terms with the hurt I caused to myself and others as I uselessly attempted to fit square pegs into round holes. It turned out I did not have to live how I had been living. I no longer scream at anyone or hurl good chocolate at the wall. I sit on the bus and *try* to think, *It's wonderful we all get to listen to this horrible music; it'll make leaving the bus and hearing police sirens and traffic all the sweeter.*

For me, ADHD is not 'special', it's not a superpower and it doesn't make you more or less intelligent than someone who doesn't have it. It is a different way that some minds work, which the world has been ignorant about accommodating until very recently.

The first time I ever heard of ADHD was in my late teens. It was mentioned in the context of boys misbehaving, being antisocial and disruptive in class, which I was not. I remember conversations and articles in which people questioned its legitimacy as a condition. There was stigma attached to not being 'normal' back then. I am from a generation where, when I was at school, any issue to do with your brain was still taboo. Offensive terms, such as 'remedial' and 'retarded', 'slow' and 'backward' were still commonly used. I did not want to be called such things and so I couldn't admit the problems I was having with my focus, which were massively impacting my ability to study. In any case, I was always too deeply locked in daydreaming or frustration to get it together to ask for help, even if help had been available. Lack of knowledge and understanding around neurodivergence is why so many in my generation and preceding ones were left undiagnosed. Undiagnosed ADHD, for me, contributed hugely to my low self-esteem, anger issues, addiction, loss of friendships, toxic and chaotic relationships, extremely messy rooms and many unfinished upcycling projects.

So what is this fancy label that I have? ADHD means your brain has a deficiency in its neurotransmitters, particularly dopamine and norephedrine, and this really messes with your executive functions, so concentration often becomes an impossible struggle and impulsive behaviour unavoidable. Put in the simplest terms, the area of the brain which controls impulsive behaviour and helps the brain organise and process stuff gets sleepy and can't be arsed doing its job properly. (I appreciate 'stuff' and 'arsed' are intimidating scientific terms. I will try not to swamp you with too much jargon.) The condition makes four key parts of your brain wander off when you want it to pay attention and process your thoughts and feelings. (ALL parts of the brain are key though, I imagine? I have never heard of a 'take it or leave it' section of grey matter, but then I learned everything I know about the human brain from Pixar's *Inside Out*.)

Those four parts are:

Frontal cortex

Possibly the most famous part of the brain, which even I had heard of. It organises the rest of your brain, controls your attention and executive function – the ability to plan, focus, multitask, exert self-control …

Limbic system

This is the deep, dark part of your brain. It processes emotions and so it is very, very important, unless you are a Vulcan.

Basal ganglia

Incredibly, not a pasta dish, but a very important component of your brain and critical in keeping other parts of your brain communicating. If they are not, you can lose concentration or impulsively jump on a trampoline WHEN YOUR IS BABY ON IT (see chapter 8).

RAS (The reticular activating system. As if you didn't know!)

This is a busy bunch of neurons that carry messages to the correct department of your brain. They are a filter system, designed to identify the important stuff and chuck out the nonsense. When it is impaired, as it is in ADHD brains, messages can scramble or not get through. Focus can be lost because your brain cannot see the bigger picture. It craves stimulation NOW to stay awake and alert, so if you are at, say, after-work drinks at a new job and conversations are very surface-level and unstimulating, and you are a bit nervous, your RAS can short circuit and you might sudden blurt out something like, 'I've been to this pub before! I've had sex in the toilets!' A non-ADHD brain prunes defunct neurons in your RAS but an ADHD brain doesn't do this effectively, so they can end up bouncing around, sending the wrong messages, creating havoc and oversharing.

So that's a snapshot of what is likely going on inside an ADHD brain. How that manifests out in the world will be different for different people. Here is a list of symptoms I had:

- Impulsiveness/not thinking of consequences
- Compulsive behaviour
- Chronic boredom (my body physically reacts to boredom. If I can't leave the room I am in, I doodle, and if I can't doodle, I claw at my flesh or consider faking my own death)
- An inability to keep physically still
- Chronic forgetfulness
- Distracted to the point where I am unable to follow conversations or instructions
- Interrupting conversations repeatedly (I promise I am otherwise a very polite and respectful person and not simply an arse)
- Not being able to start tasks
- Not being able to finish projects

- An inability to tidy up (not an excuse. I can dedicate hours to tidying up and still finish in a mess)
- Getting locked in rumination or repetitive negative thoughts
- Getting stuck in daydreams
- Hypersensitivity (if you can't regulate emotions properly it might feel like a work colleague hates you and wants you dead because they didn't return your smile, when really they have stuff on their mind other than you and didn't register it).

There are more, but you get the gist.

The origins of ADHD are debated: some suggest it's a throwback to when we were hunter-gatherers and that our ancestors with ADHD were better nourished because they were better at thinking on their feet and taking risks, like hurling themselves at those who were after their food. Once we didn't need to hunt animals and gather our food anymore, human life would have become more ordered, more linear, and those with ADHD might have struggled with this. Perhaps we became the chaos fighting back against routine and monotony? No wonder so many writers and artists have ADHD.

By the by, ADHD impulsivity and 'not thinking of the consequences of actions' is not an excuse to be an utter bastard. ADHD does not impair empathy or moral values, so if you have been a bastard, own it and get the support you need. Not everyone has the resources or the wherewithal to do this, I know, but I don't want you to think I consider ADHD an excuse to shoplift, punch people, cheat on your partner or buy a budgie just because you happened to pass a pet shop.

Also, if I may suddenly and without warning jump to another subject (I have ADHD, did I not mention it?), I don't like the term ADHD. Not because I don't want a 'label'. I have no problem with labels to describe a condition I have. For example, being labelled 'short-sighted' is fine. I do not resist going for a sight test and getting glasses because 'not being able to see when I'm driving will NOT define me!' My problem with the label is that it's not accurate.

Take the 'attention deficit' part for example. I *can* pay attention; I have plenty of focus. I have *hyper*focus, but I cannot direct my focus at will. When I'm meant to be doing something important, like my work, or a tax return, or hanging out the washing because we have all run out of clean socks, I will spend hours reading about Victorian workhouses instead. When I have an important deadline, I will idle on Twitter for hours or learn old music hall songs. 'We had to move away 'cause the rent we couldn't pay. The moving van came round just after dark.' Yes, that's right, I know the verses to 'My Old Man Said Follow the Van', 'Where Did You Get That Hat?', 'Daddy Wouldn't Buy Me a Bow-Wow' and many, many more. I do not know when my car tax is due for renewal though. The issue is that when and where I direct my focus is not in my own hands. Or, to be more accurate, in my own brain. My hyperfocus happens when I am in the last chance saloon with a deadline. When I am right at the edge, in real danger of falling, I will save myself, but not before.

This hyperfocused, heightened alertness also happens when I am on stage. I am a stand-up comedian. I have to think on my feet; I have to hold my focus; stay in the moment. Many people do not find getting up alone on stage in front of a load of strangers and trying to make them laugh particularly appealing. I, however, need extremes to be jolted out of my ADHD fog.

The 'hyperactivity' part is true, but it's usually thought of as loud and destructive, which is why it is often associated with boys who run around being 'naughty' and setting off fire alarms. But hyperactivity can be very quiet and often missed, especially in girls, who are just labelled 'a dreamer'. My form of hyperactivity was frequent and debilitating rumination, or going deep into daydreaming so I completely missed what was going on around me. (I once missed three buses in a row, while standing at the bus stop.)

When I am excited, or nervous, or overstimulated, I can talk non-stop, right over other people. I have a motor I cannot switch off. It can make me seem rude or impatient, and I *am* rude or impatient sometimes, but more often, I fall into a swirl of thoughts and responses that bubble up and I have to get out then and there. They can overwhelm me. Many people who experience this, misuse alcohol and/or drugs, or develop food compulsions and obsessive-compulsive behaviours, because without realising it they are self-medicating, finding ways to shut that motor up for a bit.

And as for the 'disorder' part, I do not believe I have a disorder. It is our disordered world that cannot accommodate brains that might work just a little bit differently.

ADHD has been described as having its 'moment' in the last few years. This just means that we have become more aware of how brains work differently, realising that one size does not fit all in education and the workplace. People like me, whose brain wanders off to dance in the woods, are beginning to understand that there is nothing *wrong* with us; it's a lack of understanding of different types of brains that shuts us out and make us feel like failures, because we are unable to do things that other people seem to find so easy.

You may have a friend, family member, partner who infuriates you because they are smart and manage some things perfectly well but they frequently lock themselves out of the house, miss appointments, constantly jump from one topic of conversation to another, interrupt, blurt out inappropriate things, can't do admin, have a wildly unpredictable temper, can't keep time, can't sit still, are an utterly impulsive flibbertigibbet. Perhaps they did incredibly well at school then unravelled at university, when the scaffolding of formal schooling and parental presence came down. Or they have 17 degrees but can't get it together to actually get a job. Maybe you know a child who seems bright but absolutely can't keep up with school work and struggles to follow tasks or understand instructions. Or people who can't keep eye contact, or can't stop talking, or seem to be utterly locked in daydreams? If you suggest they may have ADHD, might they say something like, 'ADHD? No, why do you think that? Maltipoos are my favourite cross-breed. Caroline's brother has ADHD. God, what this government is doing to opera is a disgrace. Have you seen the woman who works in the Co-op? She looks just like Ricky Gervais.'

I am not saying that everyone who does any of these things from time to time definitely has ADHD. It could be that at uni they discovered weed and sex and couldn't be arsed with studying much. Or they could be just annoying. *Or* they could have ADHD and find it incredibly frustrating that people think they are annoying or can't be arsed.

ADHD does not itself lead to poor mental health, but undiagnosed ADHD can create low self-esteem because nobody, not even you, can understand why you can't learn in the way you are expected to, why you can't manage your emotions, why you just can't 'PAY ATTENTION!'. You spend your life masking your difficulties. You cannot process your shame and frustration, so it just grows and grows.

My diagnosis in 2021 meant I got an explanation for why so many things that seemed easy enough for other people were impossible for me. Reading non-fiction (unless it's autobiographical like this book!), for example, time management, planning, self-control, tidying up, starting tasks, finishing tasks, organising, not crying and having a near-panic attack when your online banking glitches, impulsive decisions and purchases (I have 23 rolls of turquoise laminate if anyone needs it) and plain old concentration.

If you don't have ADHD you may be thinking, *Oh come on! We ALL cry down the phone to our bank sometimes and buy a llama online after a few drinks. It doesn't mean you have ADHD!* Of course it doesn't. ADHD-like symptoms can appear now and then for anyone. That's why it's easy to miss, and easy to mask. It's why it has taken so long to get its 'moment'.

When I first talked about my diagnosis on social media during the Covid-19 lockdown, I expected a little eye-rolling and comments along the lines of 'everybody wants to have *something* these days'. But that is not what happened. I was inundated with direct and public messages, many begging me to tell them where and how I got my diagnosis. They were mostly from women my age, though I also got many messages from men and from young people who told me how they had been frustrated and full of anxiety for years. Others who had already been diagnosed wrote to me, sharing their own story of relief when they got some answers to behaviours they had battled with their whole lives.

I wrote back to as many as I could, staggered that all this time, all of my 47 years, I had not been alone. I was not an outsider weirdo who was different to everyone else, as I had sometimes suspected. There were hundreds of other people who had been struggling the same way and none of us knew how common the condition was. I carried decades of shame around my inability to focus, about ways that I had acted because I couldn't navigate my emotions. I had become the butt of jokes for my disorganisation and untidiness. Labelled a space cadet, scatter brain, dipstick and told, 'You are not bringing a llama into this house!' Teachers, parents, friends, boyfriends, employers had seen my potential and couldn't understand why I insisted on messing things up.

Now, every time I do a gig, audience members come up to me afterwards to talk about ADHD. They tell me they have it or suspect they have it. One woman told me that her child was intelligent, curious, but simply could not concentrate and do her homework or revise. She was not frustrated with her daughter; she wanted to find out how to help her. This made me cry; good tears. However much this child was struggling, it was incredible to hear her parent recognise that it was not the *fault* of her child.

These messages, these conversations are why I wanted to write this book. I am not a doctor; I have not studied psychiatry, so the only advice I can give to parents who talk to me about their children is make sure your child knows that there is nothing, absolutely *nothing* wrong with them. It's just that our world hasn't bent enough yet to accommodate the different way their brain works.

I am very much behind on the deadline. I assured everyone I could write this book in six months, thinking *Yes, I have a full-on stand-up comedy tour planned, two children, elderly parents, commercial commitments, radio and television bookings … and ADHD. Sure! Six months, no problem!*

Procrastination is the most relatable symptom of ADHD and the one most likely to make people go, 'Oh I do that all the time!' Do you? To the point where you can't leave your house? Do you get court orders and fines because you procrastinate, because you can't open your post? Do you feel like your world is crashing down on you and you will lose your home because you are glued to your phone looking at pornography or looking up 'dog and cat cuddling' (porn for some, I imagine) for five hours at a time, utterly unable to get on with your work? Well then, please understand that if you have ADHD, things get more debilitating than getting a bit sidetracked.

There was a point at which my publishers got very worried. When I got off the phone to them, I pledged to myself, I actually said out loud, 'I will do nothing but write today.' And then got on the internet, drove to Greenford and bought a puppy.

Here are some other things I have done in the last few months as the deadline of this book loomed:

- Upcycled my wardrobe doors with stick-on vinyl wallpaper (saves a fortune, eats your time)
- Got a puppy
- Watched hours of 'How to groom your Maltese' videos on YouTube
- Taken a carpentry course and learned to make a shelf with brackets
- Got a certificate in psychotherapy
- Applied for a master's degree in psychotherapy
- Upcycled an art deco dressing table
- Made a table out of an old cable reel
- Written a play
- Taken a French class
- Played PAC-MAN until I was seasick

- Upcycled an old doll's house
- Been to see the Sistine Chapel.

My last minute hyperfocus means you are able to read this book now. I do get things done, just not on time, and in my own way.

This book is a look back on my life when I did not know I had ADHD. Now that I do know, I have had to look back over areas of my life – particularly my education, my relationships, parenting, my compulsions, my career – through a new lens, which has been both cathartic and very painful. So this book is laid out in thematic chapters for this reason, and also because 'structure is your Achilles heel' (the very true words of my first-ever publisher). Before I forced myself to stick to themes, I wandered endlessly off topic, into unrelated anecdotes, and we estimated I'd still be on chapter one in 2047.

I am on medication now for ADHD. I take an amphetamine that wakes up the sleepy part of my brain, the one that organises the rest of it. I am not 'cured'. There is no cure for ADHD. I still procrastinate (I know all the lyrics to all of Meghan Trainor's songs) and, most recently, I turned up a month early to a friend's book launch and a week early to my own gig. But I am much better at pre-empting mistakes and behaviours so these things happen less often, and I do not punish myself when they do. I am not flooded with shame and frustration.

Medication helps me sort through my thoughts, but it was not the pills alone that freed me from the knots of anxiety I had been tied up in for most of my life. Medicating the symptoms of ADHD is not enough to help someone. If a child, for example, shows symptoms of ADHD, thinking that a prescription of pills is the immediate solution can lead to a dangerous road. ADHD can be hereditary, but trauma can also be a contributing factor. The whole picture of a person's life needs to be taken into account to figure out why they cannot concentrate, keep still or stop talking, or why they may live in a daydream.

Talking therapy, being in nature, exercising, and learning about my brain have been crucial in managing my ADHD. Finally I understand that my mind settles when I give myself a breather in the open air instead of loading my life with more and more chores and activities, which I have always been driven to do. Now that I know I have ADHD, if anyone makes the mistake of calling me Scatty Shappi I forget to invite them to the pub.

So, are we clear? This is not a self-help book. I have no medical qualifications. I wanted to write this book about my experience because of the avalanche of people who contacted me to share their stories of late diagnosis of ADHD or were still living their life thinking, *What is wrong with me?* If any of it resonates with you, I have included some useful resources at the end. If none of it does, well, aren't you the neurotypical one?! Enjoy my chaos and luxuriate in your impeccably ordered bookcase.

Everything in this book is my own personal experience. I am not an expert; I'm a little Black woman in a big silver box. (That's a line from *Jumpin' Jack Flash*. Forgive me. I have ADHD.)

So, you are free to read this book now. I hope you enjoy it. For God's sake, finish it.

A NERD WITHOUT PORTFOLIO

'You are not stupid, are you?' Ah! The 1980s! The era when teachers were finally banned from physically assaulting children but could still heap shame on them without being questioned. Strangely, when teachers asked this of me, it didn't make me more able to keep up in class, finish my tasks or stop me daydreaming.

I was not stupid, I knew that. I read constantly; I tore through books from the library. I was articulate and well behaved and was really good at English, French and sociology. But I knew there was something up with me. I couldn't concentrate in class. I often had to fight sleep and despite my best intentions, despite swearing I would do my homework the moment I got home, I never did.

Most of my friends were in the 'accelerated learning' class, while I was often put in the lower classes with the kids who mucked about and didn't seem to care if they passed their GCSEs or not. I felt out of place there. I wasn't like them. I was a nerd who just didn't have the grades to match their interests. I was a Nerd Without Portfolio.

The teachers had a tough time accommodating me within the streaming system at my school. 'She seems to be top of the class in English and French but an absolute thicko in everything else,' I imagine they said. The highest stream was one, and the lowest was eight, and where we were put was based on an exam we sat at the end of primary school, which I only now have twigged was the eleven-plus.

Let me tell you how I did in that exam. There was a maths question that showed a circle and the instruction read: Divide this circle into six EQUAL parts.

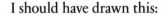

I drew this: I should have drawn this:

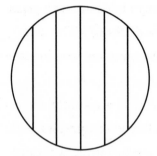 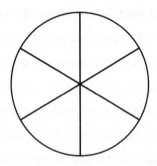

I know now that my circle does not have equal parts. I had no clue how important these tests were. I had not been prepared and I had not read the question properly. I did not think it through.

'But if you were smart then how come you never did any work and couldn't understand even the most basic maths?' I hear you ask. How did I know there was something 'wrong' rather than 'I'm just too thick to get it'? It was like being locked out of a room. As if I'd been pushed out of the room and was peering in through a keyhole. (That's a lie. I'd never have peered through the keyhole, I'd have wandered off into a dream world where Zammo from *Grange Hill* was in love with me.) It wasn't that I didn't understand the teachers' explanations – I couldn't hear them. My mind checked out. *Tralalalala!* Off it skipped into the fog with its fingers in its ears. If I was thick I wouldn't have understood my English lessons or hung back to ask my sociology teacher to tell me more about nature versus nurture. (A girl was raised in a *chicken coop! She behaved like a chicken!* This was fascinating; why couldn't we do sociology all day? If Pythagoras had been raised by chickens, or if we were taught who he actually was and what he got up to when he wasn't obsessing about triangles, I might have actually passed my maths GCSE.)

Maths, I have learned since having children who love the subject, is a language and it can't be taught in the same way to everyone. Of course, I can't tell you if this is simply to do with ADHD or if I am simply incapable of understanding maths, but when someone tries to explain a maths formula to me, it's as though they are talking to me in Mandarin (a language I do not speak). I was utterly lost from the very start. Imagine – if you can't speak Mandarin – that someone reads you a poem in Mandarin. Then they say, 'Did you understand that?' and you say, 'No.' Then they say, impatiently, 'Well, which bit didn't you understand? Everyone else got it, so why didn't you?' That was what maths was like for me throughout my school years, and it's unsurprising that it knocks the old self-esteem when you can't speak Mandarin (or maths in my case).

My focus was intense in subjects I liked, though. English, history, sociology, French – all of that was riveting. I never fought an urge to fall asleep. There was no drama class at my school. I could really have done with this – a subject in which I could do my own thing, go by my own rules. Unfortunately, my brain simply cannot stay in its seat if it is not utterly fascinated by what's going on. The slightest bit of boredom and my concentration wriggles away from me like a toddler wriggles out of someone's arms to dash off and play. I can no more command my brain to focus on something it doesn't want to than a puppy can learn to tie shoelaces: 'If only it paid attention! Come on, puppy! I *just* showed you how to tie them! Which bit didn't you get?'

I kept very quiet about the fact my brain didn't seem to be able to stay put and focus. It just couldn't. If any other part of me didn't work the way it was expected to, you could see it, but we're expected to be in control of our own brains – unless there's something 'wrong' with you. This was an era where the word 'retarded' was liberally used and the last thing you wanted to do was let on that you had any kind of difficulty with learning. Learning difficulties were what kids in 'special' schools had. Whenever teachers pulled me up on not doing homework or not paying attention, I filled up with shame. That shame built a tower of anxiety inside me and made itself at home. Neither was going anywhere for a long, long time.

My daughter was six years old at the start of the Covid-19 lockdown, when we had to home school. You'd think I'd be able to help a child of six with her maths. I could not. She watched me get a sum wrong and thought I was mucking around. She realised I wasn't when a big fat tear plopped out of my eye. She ran to get her big brother, who came down and helped his sister with her work and made me a cup of tea. All the shame, all the anxiety had come right back. Both my children enjoy maths and I have always done my best to hide the fact that I can't do it from them. Now they knew. It was like finding out their mother can't read.

'It's okay, Mama,' my daughter cooed. 'I'll teach you.'

It was time to come clean. 'You can't, darling,' I told her. 'Mummy's brain can't do maths. I can't concentrate. Not even for a minute.'

Her 12-year-old brother gently explained, 'Mummy's good at other things. She just doesn't do maths.'

My little girl consoled me with a hug. 'You are really good at doing voices.' And I am.

Where were my parents in all of this? There is a stereotype that Iranian parents are pushy about education and insist their children become doctors, lawyers, engineers or professional wrestlers. My parents are artistic people – my father is a poet and my mum was a teacher in Iran; in England she sung her heart out all day looking after us and looking after the endless stream of guests coming to our home. And they are both very smart at maths and science too. They couldn't understand why both my brother and I struggled with these things, but they were not hell-bent on us getting PhDs. We were expected to go to university and study something or other, but other than that, they were happy that my school reports all said I was a 'kind, pleasant member of the class'. This generally means 'she is not very bright but gives us no trouble', but my parents, not being au fait with the British education system, had no idea.

My parents thought that because I read a lot, I must be doing fine at school. At parents' evenings, they were told that I was 'no trouble', 'very polite', and everyone was happy. My methods worked; everyone was fooled. I thought hiding the fact that I was struggling was the 'win' rather than getting help. Not that there was anywhere to get help.

My older brother, Peyvand, took the heat off me quite a bit too by making sure teachers were in constant contact with my parents about his behaviour at school. He found school intolerable and so tended to run away from the gates from time to time. When he was there, he would do Tarzan impressions in class, often while standing on a desk. I remember his school report saying 'Peyvand thinks his entire role at school is to make his classmates laugh.' A very noble endeavour, in my book. Sadly, my parents did not see it like this and he got into trouble for being in trouble.

I understood Peyvand, though. It pained me to see how he was a square peg that adults were trying to force into a round hole. He was talented in art, really brilliant in school plays and, like me, good at French. I feel sad for him because he was labelled 'trouble' when he was a clever, bored, frustrated kid. There was nothing wrong with him; the problem was with the system which did not accommodate children who sometimes needed to beat their chest and go *ARGHAAAAAAA …ARGHAAAAAAA!* in geography class.

My mother held the firm belief that I was an academic genius. (She also thought I was an incredible gymnast due to my admittedly well-executed roly-polys, and a gifted singer, due to my rendition of 'Baa, Baa, Black Sheep' to dinner guests when I was five.) One parents' evening, my science teacher, trying to find something positive to say, told her, 'Shaparak draws very neat Bunsen burners.' That was all my mother needed to be convinced her daughter would be the first Iranian to walk on the moon. To this day, she will tell people, 'Shaparak was brilliant at science!' But I was absolutely not.

'MATHS WILL BE RELEVANT IN ANY CAREER YOU CHOOSE' came the tyrannical, relentless mantra from teachers, parents and other adults, who did not seem to understand that kids like me were neither bad on purpose nor pretending to struggle but in fact doing complicated algebra by torchlight under our duvets at night – for fun! I thought, being a stand-up, I had proved the 'IN ANY CAREER YOU CHOOSE' tyrants wrong. And for 20 years, I was triumphant. Never have I been heckled with 'Oi! I paid to find out how many apples Janet has when she starts off with 20 but gives 13 of them to Susan! ALL you're doing is JOKES! GET OFF! BOOOOOOOO!'

But then, in 2017, I found myself in a smelly, stagnant lake in the Australian jungle on the reality TV show *I'm a Celebrity … Get Me Out of Here!* (If you don't know it, it's a reality TV show where highly intelligent, humble people of note sit around discussing philosophy and occasionally doing a fun little task, like writhing in a box of snakes, in order to win food.) In the lake were giant inflatables with three- or four-figure prices on and you had to swim around in the disgusting, freezing water to find the numbers you needed to make up the sum on a giant board. There was no way I could do this, certainly not under pressure and with water snakes swimming around in my shorts. There I was, in my forties, on one of the biggest TV shows in the country, feeling like the class dunce with the other contestants shouting at me to hurry up with the impossible mental arithmetic. So it was true. Maths, and perhaps water snakes, will be relevant in any career you choose.

I have a knack of making friends with swots and misfits. This has been an unconscious survival tool. At school, it is the nice, swotty kids who will tell you what class you are meant to be in and what page you are meant to be on, and who will gently nudge you when you nod off. (Falling asleep when your brain is not stimulated enough is an ADHD trait. Which is yet another thing I now know explains a lot.) If someone is a swot *and* a misfit then it's the perfect combination, because misfits will let anyone hang out with them.

I got picked on at school by the mouthy kids because I sounded 'posh', was a bit fat and had big hair. It bewildered me, so I cocooned myself within the nerds. My nerdy friends were the reason my education did not completely sink. They unwittingly helped me mask my ADHD. They helped me with my homework on the bus on the way to school and whispered the teacher's instructions I had not been listening to. This meant I kept my head just above water and avoided being put in the very lowest bands with the girls who grew their nails to make them weapons for fights. In my little group of outcasts, I tried to have fun and look like I didn't care that I wasn't able to keep up with them academically. I did impersonations of the teachers and took the mickey out of myself – 'Hahaha! Look at me! I'm such an idiot!'

At home too, I made my parents and brother laugh by making fun of myself, of how I got things wrong at school. My brother read my essays out phonetically, with all my spelling mistakes (I am dyslexic) and we would cry laughing. I was endlessly upbeat about my low marks; I entertained my parents into not worrying about me. As long as I was making them laugh, I could keep failing at school.

My ex-husband, Christian, was the first person to call out this playing-the-fool masking that had become natural to me. It was before we got together. We were both performing at Jongleurs comedy club in Edinburgh and we had stayed behind for the disco and danced to the *Grease* medley because we were only 30 and back then, the live comedy scene was still a very boozy, *well-a-well-a-well-a-HUH* type of place.

This was 2004 and I had been on the circuit for about eight years. Learning how to do well on stage was nerve-racking, but offstage was stressful too. Being around other comedians was hard for me. They were mostly blokes back then. ADHD is no help whatsoever when you are feeling socially awkward. I was either completely silent around all the male comedians, who seemed to be so rambunctious and sure of themselves, or I would get horribly drunk. I had no pals, not proper ones at least, and so many unspoken, unprocessed feelings that I could not verbalise even to myself rampaged through me. I couldn't connect with the male comedians.

But I did connect with Christian. After the disco, we talked and walked back to the hotel together in the early hours. I felt at ease; comfortable, not the way I was used to feeling around guys. He suddenly asked me, 'Why do you pretend to be less intelligent than you are?'

Whoa. I was not prepared for realness. It stopped me in my tracks. No one had ever noticed before, or they just hadn't mentioned it – or, let's face it, didn't think it.

'Ditzy' was a persona I had developed as a way to mask how ashamed I was of the massive gaps in my education, of not always keeping up with what was going on around me. So battered was my confidence from being cast aside as a no-hoper, I announced it before more people could accuse me of it. 'Haha! Look at me! I'm crap at everything!' Far from making me friends, this defence mechanism of mine put a barrier between me and other people, with whom, if I'd been honest, I would have liked to have made a connection with – but that required an emotional unlocking that I had yet to learn to do.

We had to write an acrostic poem at primary school, using our first names. I still remember mine. It was:

Soppy's a word to describe me,
Human I am not,
Absolutely barmy
Perfectly gone to pot,
Aggravating in every way,
Rubbish at everything,

Annoying you could say
Kerfuffle I often make.

So, reading between the lines, I think it's fair to say my self-esteem issues went back a long way. At the time, I would have imagined this poem was funny. But a kid calling herself aggravating, rubbish and annoying – there is no humour here. This was a cry for help. If either of my children had ever come home with a poem like this about themselves, I would drop everything to support them to build up their self-esteem, until they were running through the streets singing 'This Is Me' from *The Greatest Showman* with all their heart and soul. But the 1980s was a different time.

I remember my parents disliking the 'rubbish at everything' line and my mother saying something along the lines of 'you are not rubbish, you draw very nice Bunsen burners', but no one investigated deeper. I recognise that I am a parent in very different times and circumstances. I have had slightly different problems as a parent than my own had. My folks were raising two young children in exile while their family in Iran were plunged into a war with Iraq. My mother would be thinking, *I wonder if my family survived last night's air raid* as she got us ready for school while today I might think, *I wonder if they got my joke on the class WhatsApp group? It only got two laugh emojis.*

My parents' concerns were 'Have we enough money for the rent?' and 'Is there a bomb under the car?' They didn't have the headspace I do of being able to sit my child down and say, 'How did it make you feel when Toby called you a bogey-head?'. But back in the 1980s, there was no talk of self-love or self-worth, and children were often left free to be endlessly negative about themselves.

In our school's streaming system, band one was the top class and band eight was the bottom class. I was put in bands four and five for maths and science, so the best the timetable would allow for French and English was band two. Bands seven and eight were for the children in the LS group. LS stood for Learning Support. The only time we all mixed was when we did games. (Why did they decide PE was the place to suddenly become egalitarian? I wish there had been bands for PE.)

- Monday: Scary sporty types who jump over you as you lie down exhausted.
- Tuesday: Wholesome all-rounders who aren't team leaders but are always the first to be picked.
- Wednesday: Those who can't catch but can run 100m without passing out.
- Thursday: The daydreamers who don't understand the rules but will wander around doing the occasional cartwheel.
- Friday: Those who can just about manage a walk around the field while eating crisps.

(I'd be in Thursday's group.)

I got the bus to and from school with one of the girls in the LS group. I couldn't understand why she was in the LS class, so I asked her (because I have ADHD and tact is something I have had to work on over the years). Denise was her name. She shrugged and said, 'They think I'm thick.'

'Oh,' I said.

Her acceptance of this was heartbreaking.

Maybe she had ADHD or another kind of neurodivergence and couldn't mask it like I did? Maybe her mum didn't tell her she was a genius at everything like mine did, so she believed it when she was treated as though she was 'thick'. Maybe she came from a long line of people who were neurodivergent in some way but didn't know and they all believed 'we're all just thick' so she accepted it as normal, the way the child of a circus acrobat might accept that balancing on their mum's head then triple somersaulting onto their dad's hands before they all sit down to lunch is normal.

There were so many kids at my school from what we would now call 'challenging' backgrounds, but back then we called 'rough'. The lower the band the school's streaming system put you in, the rowdier the kids that were your classmates. I was terrified of a lot of the kids I had to sit in class with, which, to be honest, didn't help. Sometimes lessons were just 45 minutes of the teacher trying to stop kids from talking, fighting and jumping on tables. I didn't have a prayer of processing all the new people, new experiences. It was all a noisy, intimidating, unfathomable battleground.

I had learned at a very young age that speaking 'like the Queen' meant that teachers liked you and were far more likely to believe your lies about why you hadn't done your homework, than if you spoke more 'cockney'. Accents are, to an extent, a choice. In a school where the kids who were struggling mostly had working-class accents, I adopted a very middle-class one. My parents would get the odd 'bloody foreigners' hurled at them when we were out and about, so when I was little, I consciously spoke 'posh' because I was scared of racists and a P*ki kid (what I was often called in the 1970s and 1980s) speaking the Queen's English placated them.

At secondary school, many middle-class kids did the opposite: they made their accents more cockney to fit in. But I couldn't because I knew a posh accent made my excuses for not doing work more believable. Also, I could escape to the welfare room and miss classes if I couldn't face a bully or just hadn't done my work. 'I'm so sorry, I'm feeling quite sick' in a middle-class accent was rarely questioned.

The down side of this was that I fooled the other children too, who couldn't imagine that I hadn't done my homework. 'Oi! Posh swot! Let me copy your homework.'

'I haven't done it,' I'd say, cheeks burning.

'Liar!' they'd say, and throw my bag across the room.

I was not a liar. I was not the swot they thought I was. I never did my homework. Ever. I couldn't. I imagine I'd have got my head kicked in if I said in my Jeeves voice, 'Now, now, old chap, no call for that. I, like you, am a total dunce! Haven't done a jot of homework and never will. What say we bury the hatchet and I'll keep lookout while you set off the fire alarm?' So I kept my head down and counted the minutes and seconds until we were free to go home.

The main lesson I learned at school was to hide the fact that I was learning nothing. I studied How To Be Invisible in Class rather than the Russian Revolution. (My 15-year-old son is currently learning about the Russian Revolution. He loves it. He chats to me about all the key characters. Laa-Laa, Tinky-Winky and Po, if memory serves me correctly.) I hid my exercise books and pretended I had lost them so teachers wouldn't see the empty pages. I was ashamed of my secret of being unable to focus. I had heard the way people spoke about the kids in the bottom classes. They were seen as different from everyone else; mentally defective. I couldn't have anyone think that of me, though I needed the same support that they were getting.

Homework was impossible, even with the subjects I liked. I don't mean I found it hard; I mean I couldn't even start it. Starting things was impossible. I took my books home and when I tried to get on with it, my brain would not cooperate. It either fidgeted, slept or went off and did something else. I would sit and stare at my books. *I will start!* I would think. *Any minute now, I will open my book and write about Tinky-Winky!* But I never even got as far as opening my book. Sometimes I never got as far as getting my books out of my bag or even sitting at my desk. Every day was about concocting a new lie about why I hadn't done my work (Ealing buses were full of imaginary homework).

'From tomorrow', I frequently declared to myself, 'I will pay attention in class, I will be studious.' But homework remained undone and 'SHE DOES NOT WORK TO HER FULL POTENTIAL' remained the theme in all of my end-of-year reports. Because my behaviour was good in lessons and I was articulate, teachers thought my failures were down to laziness, that I didn't care. But I did care. When people shake their heads and say what a shame it is that with all your potential, if you just focus, if you just stop deliberately being rubbish just to annoy people, you could really achieve great things, you start to think, *If these smart people can't see there is a problem here, that there is a reason I can't do these things, then I must be the problem. I am, therefore, a fucking arsehole.*

Every day of my life at school was blighted by the anxiety of work I hadn't finished and tasks I did not understand because I hadn't been listening. 'What are we meant to be doing?' I asked my friends on a loop, the second the teacher finished telling us what we were meant to be doing. It was a given that to be friends with me meant that you needed to tell me what work I was meant to be doing, what class I was meant to be in and, often, what the answers were. Really, they should have been paid for the work they put in for me.

Underneath it all was a swot and nerd desperate to come out, but I just kept getting pulled into the fog. There were things I very much wanted to learn about. Gorillas, for example. And dogs and why sometimes cats eat their kittens. I wanted to know all about Horatio Nelson and his life on the sea and why he was in love with Emma Hamilton when he was married to someone else. Why did they give us lovely snippets of stories like this at school but then leave me to scour the shelves of the library in Ealing Broadway to find out more?

Overwhelmed, I would do anything to sit in the quiet and calm of the welfare room. I would stick my fingers in my throat to get something in the sick bowl they gave me. A few years later, I would become an expert at getting gallons of vomit up but, alas, at the point when I was trying to get out of classes, I was still an amateur. I would feign headaches and, before a burst vein in my nose was cauterised, I could make my nose bleed fairly easily. Blood was an instant ticket to the welfare room. I could tell the other kids were jealous. There, the kindly school nurse looked after me, gave me humbugs and I let the sweet smell of the giant bowl of diluted Dettol be my refuge away from the confusion of the classroom.

'You are turning into Shaparak the Blob!' My French teacher called me this when she asked me to stay behind for 'a little word' about my lack of focus in class. I was a bit overweight and got teased for it at school, so when my teacher selected this particular word to describe my vagueness and inattention, I was ashamed.

She was only trying to help me. I had been very good at French. When I started secondary school, the French teacher assumed one of my parents was French (which delighted my mother). Now, though, in our GCSE years, where time, structure and revision had become critical, I was totally at

a loss with all of my work. 'You are always looking out of
the window. You seem to be on another planet. Is there
something wrong?'

'I am afraid, miss, that I am unable to talk about what is
wrong. My self-esteem has been firmly hammered into the
ground at this school, where I have not found a place, or a
moment, to feel safe, to be myself. I arrived full of enthusiasm
but fell through the cracks. I am intimidated every day by the
Scary Kids and have bottled up every emotion. Every bright
spark I had has been snuffed out because all my energy has
gone into desperately trying to remain invisible, unnoticed,
because I am full of shame, full of fear. Because I cannot be
myself here. "Myself" is not acceptable here.'

That would have been my speech if this were a Netflix
series. But it is not. It was 1988, in a giant, loveless comprehen-
sive school. In reality, I just shrugged, looked at my feet and
mumbled, 'dunno miss' and that was that. The only time any
teacher tried to help me.

I passed four GCSEs. My B in French was devastating.
I should have walked an A but I had a blue Slush Puppie
on the way to school and was sick in my reading exam. To
this day, I wonder how none of the teachers, or my parents,
thought to find a way for me to resit it. I sulked about that B
for 30 years. I got 'Unclassified' for business studies because
I fell asleep – yes, really. I wrote poems in the margins of my
maths paper and got a D. (Though I upped my game when I
retook it at sixth-form college. This time, I got an E but the
poems in the margins were much better.)

I needed to get out of school and go to college. Here is where hyperfocus comes in. I bimbled along in fog and anxiety, but when right at the very edge, when I was in real danger of dropping out and not getting any more qualifications, my brain snapped into action. I took a year out and spent that year working several strange and awful jobs while I got a GCSE in Persian, bringing the total to five, so I could go to Richmond upon Thames College to do theatre studies, English and communication studies A levels.

Keeping up with this was still hard. Coursework and homework were almost impossible. But, as ever, I made friends with a very clever person, Suze. Suze was from a very posh family, had been to boarding school and didn't know what popcorn was. She was the most exotic person I had ever met. Just before our exams, Suze invited me to go with her to her mother's house in the countryside to revise for a week. I thought we were going to muck about but Suze had a STUDY PLAN. It was out of this world. She seemed to *know* how to study. We revised in the conservatory of her mother's beautiful house. It was peaceful and calm and we had no distractions. I really loved Suze; I was in awe of her and absolutely didn't want to annoy her by mucking about or chatting. She was clever and saw me as an equal to her in this respect, which is why she trusted me to come with her on a revision week and not waste the time. I could not let her down. I had never had an environment like this to work in, where there were no other distractions, where I could see a beautiful garden and hear birdsong and where there was a sweet dog asleep by my feet.

There was no risk of someone shouting or strangers coming in (to my horror, my father once invited a double-glazing salesman to join us for dinner). There was just me and Suze and our books. And I worked, without falling asleep. This was the world I wanted to belong to, to fit in with.

Suze had a strict timetable. We revised from 9am–12pm. Her mum brought us a cup of tea and a biscuit at 10.30am. Then at 12pm, we walked the dogs and had a sandwich, then it was back to work from 1pm until 4pm. It was the most ordered week of my life to date and the only reason I passed my A levels. How was I able to concentrate for those long stretches? Being away from my own chaotic home, having space somewhere calm and quiet, was a game changer. Suze broke up the study day with a walk in the woods with the dogs. Nature is critical if you suffer from the whirring overload of ADHD, I now know (though I obviously didn't put two and two together back then. Bloody maths). At home, my mealtimes were erratic and I had begun to binge eat. At Suze's mum's house, mealtimes and snack times were ordered, simple and we were not free to rummage around finding extra food.

Passing my A levels was critical. I wanted an adventurous life, I wanted to go out in the world and meet more people, to get out of Ealing where I was Shaparak the Blob, reinvent myself. Suze had a car and drove us to get our exam results from college. We had to queue. I had applied for universities. Whether or not I got to go and be the sort of person who got a *degree* depended on these A-level results. A girl in front of me in the queue was told by her French teacher, 'Michelle! You got an A!' I watched Michelle's joy as she heard that news. *Imagine*, I thought, *being someone who gets an A for their A levels*. I could only ever dream of being such a person. As I queued to look at my own results on the noticeboard I thought about how amazing it would be to be able to go home and tell your mother you had an A.

I finally got to the board. I had been predicted C-C-C and, sure enough, there was theatre studies, C; communication studies, C again ... I ran my finger along the line. English, A. Annoying. I must have looked at the wrong one. I put my finger on my name and ran it down the line again. Again it went to an A. I called to Suze (who had got three As and nodded to herself in approval). 'You look. Look at my English. Is that right?'

Suze looked and squealed, then picked me up. 'YOU GOT AN A!!!' she screamed.

I got an A! An A! ME! I was right! I was not a blob!

Look, I know I have been going on about school for a while now and, let's face it, it was quite a long time ago. But this is honestly the short version. When I first started writing this book, looking back at my life now that I know I had ADHD, for a very long time I could not stop writing about my secondary school years. On and on, for pages and pages I locked myself back into my secondary school. People in the publishing industry are a lot more tactful than in my normal comedy industry and for ages I thought everyone was absolutely fine for the entirety of my book to be about how I am still so bitterly disappointed about only getting four GCSEs. 'Um, I think your readers *may* be interested in other parts of your life too. Seventeen chapters on how you couldn't get to grips with the Corn Laws may be a *tad* too much,' I was gently informed. Whereas a comedian mate would say, 'Gawd, love, let it go. No one cares. Say something *funny*.'

But I think the reason I am struggling to let it go is that for decades my being written off at school seemed like my fault. But it wasn't. It was the fault of a system which, at the time, failed children with learning difficulties. ADHD and other neurodivergent conditions have nothing to do with your intelligence. But when I was at school, how 'smart' you were considered to be was dependent on how well you were able to fit in the system. (And 'fitting in' was also, of course, dependent on your social class and race too.)

I was in a coffee shop about five years ago when I grabbed a fancy magazine and started reading an interview with artist and film-maker Steve McQueen. I vaguely knew that he was from Ealing too, but I hadn't realised how close in age we are. He talked about how, as a dyslexic Black kid, he was written off as 'non-academic' at school, and how kids like him were expected to do a plumbing course rather than GCSEs in the arts. The way he talked about his school, the frustration, the disappointment he still clearly felt, mirrored my own feelings. I looked him up on Wikipedia. Ah, and there it was. The same school I went to, albeit a few years above me. He went on to win the Turner Prize and an Oscar; I went on to play medium-sized art centres around the country and once hosted the Loo of the Year Awards. We showed them, Steve!

I have to make something very clear: if you or a child you know has any of the problems I describe in this chapter, and indeed in this book, ADHD may well have a hand in it. But it's not enough to say, 'AHA! THAT'S what's at the bottom of it! To a psychiatrist we must go and get medication!'

As I said in my introduction, which I am sure you read thoroughly and took notes, these things are nothing without looking at the whole picture of what is going on for a child. If a kid is being brought up in a chaotic household, is dealing with trauma, has suffered a loss, then 'acts out', drifts off at school or can't keep up with work, you can't just diagnose and medicalise it as ADHD like you would athlete's foot (here's where I really hope athlete's foot is never brought on by psychological trauma – I haven't actually checked).

There is no scientific consensus, but it is generally believed that ADHD is caused by a chemical imbalance in the brain, but it is not the only reason these imbalances occur. The whole picture of a child's life needs to be looked at. The whole picture of anyone's life, who thinks they may have ADHD.

'Are you dyslexic?' was the note I got back on the first essay I wrote at King Alfred's College, Winchester (now the University of Winchester). I got a dyslexia test. I was. ADHD would have been obvious too, if anyone had known about it.

I had carried bucketloads of bitterness around my education and possessed a well of rage at the system that wrote me off.

But then a chance meeting with one of my old teachers led to my being able to lay some ghosts to rest.

From the moment I left, I avoided the part of Ealing my school was in. When I had to run past the building as part of the Ealing Half Marathon, I blew a raspberry at it. Then I bumped into Mr Houlihan (*not his real name*) in a restaurant on the Isle of Wight. He was on holiday, sitting with his family at the table next to mine. He turned to me and said, 'Do you remember me?' and I instantly did. He looked miraculously the same. Kind, sincere face, killer cheekbones.

The words that came out of my mouth immediately, 30 years on, were: 'Mr Houlihan! That school fucked me up!'

Without blinking he said, 'I know. Would you like to have a cup of tea when we are back home?' Mr Houlihan was exactly as I remembered him: very cool, sincere, a dude.

When we met up at a pub in Ealing where he still lived and I had moved back to, I poured my heart out to him about everything you have just read in this chapter. He listened and at the end, told me that the school was aware of pupils it had let down in its history.

'I want you to know', my old school teacher said, 'that you didn't "fail" at school because you have ADHD or dyslexia or because your parents couldn't navigate the system. You were let down. *We* failed you. *We* let you fall through the cracks. You have achieved so much despite that. You were *our* loss.'

He looked at me and said with calm sincerity, 'I would like you to know that I am sorry.'

Wow. I was not expecting that. I had needed to hear this without even knowing it. He could have simply listened, been sympathetic, and I would have been grateful for that. But sympathy, while soothing, doesn't heal old wounds. Empathy can though. Mr Houlihan understood this and his apology came from a place of real understanding. His apology brought me peace and I finally began to detach from this decades-old bitterness and upset from my secondary school years.

'Sorry' is a vital and beautiful word. 'Sorry' doesn't mean 'it was all my fault'. 'Sorry' can mean 'it wasn't *your* fault; the shame was not *your* burden to carry.'

Same old Mr Houlihan. There never was any small talk with him. And what a lovely thing it was to have my old school teacher buy me a beer and fish and chips – and tell me how proud he is of me. This was the closure I needed.

With his support, I went back to visit my old school – the place I had marked as the dark blot on my life. However, you can't just walk into schools these days and, to be clear, I did not just wander off the streets demanding 'TAKE ME TO YOUR LEADER!'

I rang the bell at the gate and a friendly looking man greeted me. 'What do you teach?', I asked him. 'I'm head of pastoral care', he replied.

'Wow', I said. 'We didn't have pastoral care back in my day; we just had a sick bowl.' He smiled warmly, the way nice people do when someone has just blurted out something weird.

The head teacher, the first woman in the school's history to be head, welcomed me into the place I had been dreading revisiting since the day I left. I expected to see the ghost of 13-year-old me, shuffling head bowed down the corridor with her brother's old duffle bag, while boys fought and girls shrieked. But she wasn't there. Instead, I saw children walking side by side, their heads help up. No shrieking; no barging. There were no echoing calls of 'OPEN YOUR LEGS, FERTILISE YOUR EGGS' and the atmosphere was calm and pleasant. As my son reminds me, it's not the 1980s anymore.

I sat in the head teacher's office. She listened to my tales of the school in 'those days'. It was a world away from the place we were now. We walked along the corridor to where the old science lab was. My tutor room used to be there, with a giant glass case of locusts and huge *Little Shop of Horrors*-type plants.

Nowadays, this is a school where struggling children's needs are met. Their Special Educational Needs department is not hidden away – it is situated in a beautiful glass building in the thick of it all, because stigma has been locked out. I spoke to teaching assistants who were clued up about ADHD and other neurological differences. The children chatted away cheerily to the head teacher and seemed confident and secure. In short, the school of my nightmares is now a place I'd consider setting up camp so my daughter is in the catchment area.

TUCKER JENKINS CAME FOR LUNCH (AND OTHER LIES)

I cannot play a computer game more complicated than PAC-MAN (why even bother? It is the most perfect game. I have beaten my high score on it about twenty times while I was supposed to be writing this book) and have never participated in a game of Monopoly until the end. My brain wants instant gratification. Figuring out a long-term strategy bores me to agitation. I know Monopoly is a low bar to set as an example of committing to a goal, but what can I say? I have ADHD. After the excitement of securing the top hat as my piece, I would, after a few short rounds, lose interest and start stealing from the bank, because *that* was exciting, *that* was heart-thumpingly risky. No one suspected me. Thieves are loud, naughty boys, right? Not quiet little girls.

A long-term goal does not satisfy my brain. Try telling a toddler they can't have ice cream until next year and you'll get the same level of understanding and excitement. My brain desperately looks constantly for another reward instead. Have you ever heard someone talk about the ADHD 'motor'? For me, it is always there, encouraging me to ACT ON IMPULSE! It can wake me up in the night (*Surprise! Here are all your fears and worries!*), or rugby tackle me when I need to get on with something important (*What do you mean you need to fill in a form to apply for a job? So you can get paid? Are you crazy? Let's paint the skirting board using rainbow colours instead!*). This non-stop fizzing energy makes me fidget, talk non-stop, interrupt people and move away from something without finishing it, or indeed, starting it. It makes sitting still when you are not riveted by what is going on absolute agony. My ADHD motor got more rampant and out of control as I stepped out of childhood and into adolescence. The world got more complicated and there were more uncomfortable feelings to avoid, so my motor skedaddled in all directions.

My impulsiveness has made my life exciting but also full of trouble and heartache. On the one hand, I am madly spontaneous, which can be great fun. 'YES! LET'S DO IT!' was my response to everything, for decades of my life. I was always the one at the end of the night in the pub who would say to a rabble of people I'd just met, 'PARTY BACK AT MY HOUSE!' And back these strangers would pile, eating and drinking me out of house and home, often crashing on my floor for the night. Back in the bedsit days of my twenties (and some of my thirties), drunken, chaotic nights were a way of life. I never considered how this merciless depletion of my energy, this utter lack of boundaries, often led to some kind of drama. Or how a drunken, regrettable one-night stand or a falling-out with someone, and the crushing shame of a bitter hangover as I made my way home from Dalston, might make me feel afterwards. (It was always Dalston. I'm still not sure where Dalston is exactly. I only know it's about thirty-seven bus changes back to Ealing.) I never processed, I never checked in with my own feelings. In fact, if anybody had used the phrase 'checked in with my feelings' in the 1990s, I would have thought they were tripping.

My motor never stopped. I didn't know this for decades, but much of the booze I poured down my throat – and my compulsive overeating – was me trying to shut this motor up as it rampaged through me like a quad bike driven by the Tasmanian devil. I never knew it was something that could be managed, something I could stop or redirect. I never even identified it as a 'motor' until I was diagnosed and began to experience life without it. I was just 'mad', 'ditzy', 'scatty', 'manic' and very often, I imagine (I know), a massive pain in the arse.

Looking back, the clues that this was ADHD were always there. At school, I doodled obsessively and pinched the skin on my palm, making it hurt, to get me through a boring lesson. If a teacher told me off for talking or fidgeting, I was utterly wounded. If anybody so much as looked at me with unfriendliness, it felt as though I'd been slapped. What was wrong with me? As much as I possibly could, I held all that energy inside me, the chatter building up until I became like a little pressure cooker and I did something I shouldn't, just for a split second of tension relief.

No child likes to be told off or ridiculed, but my pressure-cooker brain absolutely could not stand it. I had what is known as ADHD hypersensitivity. If I was told off, it burned me to my core, igniting a mountain of shame that had built up from all of the frustration of not fitting in, not being able to understand things the way other people did. When you are so terrified of being told off, when you know how much shame it would unearth, it makes the stakes higher.

My own childhood circumstances weren't conventional. I had a loving but often chaotic home life with parents who were dealing with exile, a revolution and then a long war in their home country. They were separated from their large families, their financial assets all seized in Iran and my father, a dissident writer, got death threats and was the target of a (foiled) assassination plot by the Iranian government. It's a wonder that I ever felt I had to make up lies to get attention.

My parents argued a lot with one another. Horrible fights, where the shouting would go on for hours and my brother and I would alternate between uselessly begging them to stop and hiding together under our beds. Children cannot understand warring adults. It creates a huge amount of stress for them to carry in their tiny bodies. And it's had a lasting affect on both my brother and me.

Like Thing One and Thing Two, cortisol – the stress hormone – rampaged through me and adrenaline blew a massive raspberry at any kind of rational thought that might be lurking, shooting it down and instead giving the command of *Fight!*, *Flight!* or *Freeze!*. It happened when I was overwhelmed, feeling shy, unable to understand a task, bored, feeling rejected, feeling anything at all. Feelings did not know where to sit. I was unable to process them. Unconsciously, I believed I must just stifle them, without thinking through the consequences. I just thought I was a weirdo and needed to hide my weirdo ways from people. I learned to mask every uncomfortable feeling. Also, if you have ADHD, your dopamine levels are lower and taking risks gives you a momentary sensory high, out of your funk, your fog, just for a moment, but I had no prayer of knowing this as a child, of course.

I did mad, stupid things all the time. Things I needed to keep secret. It might be lying; it might be stealing; it might be throwing a tin of paint onto a fire (which nearly took my face off every time I did it). I spent a lot of time unsupervised as a child and as a parent now, I stand at the door and watch if my nine-year-old pops in to our neighbour's house, to make sure she is in safely (and I do more neurotic things, like keeping rope in every bedroom in case anyone needs to climb out of the window in the middle of the night, but let's not dwell on that for now). But children weren't supervised as vigorously when I was growing up. We were all allowed, for example, as young as five and six, to play in the park next to our flat with groups of other kids of similar ages. Occasionally, a man would wander into the park in his dressing gown and try to talk to us. 'Just keep inside the playground and stay away from him,' our mums would warn. I actually think he brought parents peace of mind – 'Oh it's fine! There's a pervert in the park, he keeps an eye on the children.'

Our home was a beautifully shabby rented flat in a huge, unkempt, but very much loved (by us) Victorian house. We were the longest-residing tenants in the place. There were six flats in all, and my parents made friends with every tenant who came and went. My brother and I had free run of the house, dangling out of high windows and climbing over the garage roof to get into our huge, overgrown garden, which contained an old Victorian greenhouse, overrun by cats, and an old bomb shelter flooded with rainwater that we loved to throw bricks in. When I got older, I learned other ways to relieve the pressure that grew in my brain, but a seven-year-old has limited access to lager and bags of doughnuts.

Lots of kids lie and steal at some point and they do it for all kinds of reasons. Attention is a big one. A girl at my school told everyone she had leukaemia once. This sort of lying required research and forward planning. She came into school with her arm bandaged one day and said she'd had an operation over the weekend. Nobody believed her, although I indulged her a little because even I knew some serious stuff had to be going on for her to make something like that up. I was delighted she was my friend. She made me feel more normal.

I wasn't after the same kind of attention as her and my methods were far more spontaneous – research, forward planning and long-term commitment not being my strengths. I never, ever planned to steal; I never thought about lying in advance. What I really craved was feeling present, out of my fog. Equally, I felt an absolute horror at being told off, so I trained myself not to make a fuss, to always be seen as 'easygoing'. And yet, I jeopardised this by taking impulsive, risky gambles and telling mad lies for no real reason, such as informing everyone in my class that I knew Tucker Jenkins from *Grange Hill* and could get them all his autograph. Back then, this teen soap opera was the most popular TV show of the time. It was about a bunch of unruly kids in a secondary school and was a way of life for us 1980s kids. Tucker, the main character, the top dog, was the one a lot of the girls in my class adored, including me. One girl, Lindsay, laughed at me. 'He would never fancy YOU!'

This was rude and hurt my feelings, so naturally I said, 'Well, I know him in real life and he said he likes me as a friend but he doesn't want a girlfriend.' I did not know him in real life, obviously, and I had no idea how he felt about having a girlfriend.

'HOW do you know him?' Lindsay Galbraith asked, standing with her arms folded in a power stance, her friends on either side of her, brandishing nunchucks (I may be imagining the nunchucks).

'They were filming in our road and he came to our house for lunch.'

A good liar must have believable lies, otherwise you just look bonkers. I took pride in my lies. I could actually visualise Tucker having dinner with my parents. My parents often invited people they had just met for dinner (a very Iranian trait), so they would definitely have had Tucker Jenkins in for a meal if he had been shooting a few scenes in our road and was peckish. Suddenly everyone, including my teacher, wanted to hear about when I met Tucker. Later, my brother Peyvand helped me forge his signature from the *Grange Hill Annual*. Then more people asked for autographs.

A boy in my class named Richard Gedding (*not his real name*) could see my stress. He was the most prolific liar during my time at school. Everybody had heard his tales of his grandad owning Buckingham Palace or having to have an operation because he swallowed a kettle. I don't think he cared that nobody believed him. 'You made it up, didn't you?' he said to me one day. Not in an accusatory way, but gently and understandingly, while trying to find something he'd lost up his nose. *Oh no, Richard Gedding!* I thought. *We are not kindred spirits!* I shook Gedding off, making it clear that we were not going to bond over this.

I lived in terror that people would find out I lied. Anxiety gripped my chest every morning before school. My only solace was a fantasy that Tucker Jenkins came for a visit to our school to give a talk at our assembly, like firefighters and police officers sometimes did to tell us not to play on railway tracks or set fire to ourselves. Lindsay Galbraith would try to humiliate me and tell him, 'Shaparak said she *knows* you,' and smirk, thinking she'd rumbled me. But he would see what was going on, because he was Tucker Jenkins and he was cool. Tucker would not see me humiliated.

'Shaparak!' he'd say. 'I didn't know you went to school here! How are you?' And everyone's jaws would drop and they would go, 'WOW! We had no idea Shaparak was so cool. She really *does* know him.'

(Years later, I was commissioned to write one of Sky TV's *Little Crackers*, a short vignette from my childhood. I chose this Tucker Jenkins fantasy. The real Tucker Jenkins, the actor

Todd Carty, agreed to be in it. I got to wear a wedding dress and 'marry' him and drive away in a Ford Cortina with 'JUST MARRIED' on the back. If Todd Carty found it unnerving to be in a confined space with a woman who spent her childhood being obsessed with him, then built a career for herself which allowed her to eventually marry him on TV, he did not let it show. What a pro.)

I learned to keep my fantasies more private. My ADHD locked me into them. They weren't always romantic; sometimes I'd be rescuing kittens from a burning building. I would go so deep into the fantasy that I'd almost be in a trance. I did not grow out of them. In adulthood, reality was something to escape. If I had to apply for a job, sort out my rent, open post, off my mind would go. I know now that this was maladaptive daydreaming, quite common in people with ADHD. Later, in my teen years, my daydreams included involuntary facial expressions, murmuring and whispering that everybody seemed to notice, no matter how hard I tried to be discreet.

Lying was a performance, but impulsive stealing gave me a much-needed dopamine hit. My stealing hurt other people *and then I had to lie about it.* It filled me with deep shame, so why did I do it? What was this awful part of me? I had no clue about the chemical deficiency in my brain so, as a young child, I was horrified at this uncontrollable side of me that went, fundamentally, against the values I was raised with. I am not a sociopath (my therapist has confirmed this) so this self-inflicted humiliation and anguish baffled me. I never stole to be malicious or because I thought it was fun or because I wanted the thing I had stolen. It wasn't fun, but it was a high – a danger that did not feel good but nonetheless gave me a moment of respite from my 'motor'. My mind slowed, was in the moment, utterly focused on what I was about to do. Then afterwards, a brief euphoric adrenaline rush before the shame crashed in. Shame was never a deterrent because the compulsion was too strong, too overwhelming.

To be clear, I was not raised by the Kray twins. Stealing was completely against the morals my parents instilled in me and my brother. I once carried a box of strawberries unnoticed out of a pick-your-own field without paying for them. We were already in the car and driving away when my mum found out. Furious, she and my dad drove back and my mum marched me to the farm shop, but they had already closed. I had to leave the strawberries on the grass outside. Stolen strawberries were to be left to rot rather than consumed. She made me swear never to do such a heinous thing again. It was hardly *The Italian Job*, but my mother's disappointment taught me a serious lesson: to never, ever let her know when I had stolen something again.

My earliest memory of thieving was when I was only about six. I stole a pack of miniature pencils from a girl called Nina. Five teeny pencils from a shop in Ealing Broadway called Confiserie Française, which sold beautiful pencil cases and scented rubbers (all highly desired in the 1970s and 1980s, and on sale online now for around £100, which is a kind of robbery itself). Nina was my friend. I had been round to her house to play and had fish fingers for the first time in my life. They were the most delicious things I'd ever eaten. At my own house, we did not have such delicacies. My mother only made Persian food. Boring old slow-cooked lamb or chicken with saffron rice infused with rose water, with sprinkles of deep red barberries. Nina's mum and other mums in the school were very sweet to my own mother, who was in a new country and grappling with the language, but they never taught her to make fish fingers, sadly. Other parents saw the horrors in Iran, which we had escaped from, on the news. In their kindness, they welcomed me. In return, I stole miniature pencils from one of their children.

They were there, on the table we shared in our classroom. Everyone was doing other things; the desk was unguarded. *I could take them*, came the thought in my head. No further thoughts came. Most definitely none relating to the consequences, which were upsetting my friend and getting into trouble. But no, my brain just instructed me, quite maniacally: *TAKE THEM! TAKE THE PENCILS! TAKE THEM NOW!* So, heart pounding, I did and slipped them into the pocket of my school cardigan. Now what? NOW WHAT, BRAIN? Nothing. No answers, just panic. And guilt, and shame.

The agony of seeing Nina look for her treasured pencils did not make me confess. I just sat there, my face burning. People were looking for Nina's pencils. Nina was upset; she was crying. They were part of a set, a Christmas present. She had brought them in to show us. They were declared missing and suddenly the cry 'SHAPARAK STOLE THEM!' came from Detective Lindsay Galbraith, aged seven (she was my nemesis at school, in case I haven't made this clear enough). 'She was at the table. She must have taken them.'

There was only one thing for it. No, I did not confess. I was too scared. The disgrace and the shame would be too much to bear. I took the pencils out of my pocket and said, 'I have the same ones. They are mine, but Nina, you can have them. Don't cry. You can have my ones.' I gave Nina her own pencils back. I was praised by our teacher for my kind generosity and Lindsay Galbraith was told off for 'accusing Shaparak without any proof'. Not only had I stolen and upset my friend, but I managed to get law-abiding, if bloody annoying, Lindsay a telling-off for rightly accusing me of stealing.

A couple of boys at my school did more overtly antisocial stuff, which the teachers had to deal with. One boy used to take his willy out in class all the time. Another boy used to get so angry in class that he once threw his chair at the teacher. Our teacher stayed calm and another teacher who heard the shouting came in and ushered us all out. We heard the boy still screaming. Other teachers came out; his parents were called. The atmosphere amongst us children was of concern, sadness even. The kid was a nice boy. It was clear, even to us children, that there was something wrong. He had some time off school and when he came back, he was not in trouble. He was given space. He took some classes with a 'special teacher', one-on-one. I don't know if these boys were neurodivergent. I don't know what was going on for them. I do know that they were not 'bad' kids; I could see the teachers deploying a kind of care towards them that was different to the way they dealt with ordinary naughty behaviour. I related to the boy who threw the chair (not so much to the boy who got his willy out). I felt like I was throwing chairs around too, but on the inside.

One day, in the last year of primary school, my thieving escalated. I did not plan it. I walked to the loos at school, past the coats, trustingly hung up on racks. I did not want to leave this school. I was at home here. The secondary school I was going to, and had visited, was huge and very daunting. I was terrified but it would not have occurred to me to tell anybody this.

I put my hand in the pocket of one of the coats. I wasn't looking for anything. But I touched cold metal. A 50-pence piece. I took it and felt an instant high. But later, when it was too late to put it back, that was replaced with shame, regret and despair. When the owner of the coat, Julie, discovered her bus money had gone, she stood in the corridor and sobbed. How could I give it back to her without getting into trouble? I couldn't. I just watched as teachers came to her aid and arrangements were made to get her home.

Whenever I took something, my heart beat fast: I had a very real, actual moment where I felt something intense. At home I stole my dad's cigarettes. Right from under his nose. It helped that his desk was utterly chaotic, absolutely covered with paper, books, pens, empty glasses of tea and shot glasses. I would chat to him while he was absorbed in his writing and only half listening, quickly swipe a cigarette, then leave him alone. Smoking it out of the bathroom window was another heart-thumping risk.

A darker way to calm down my 'motor' was to strangle myself (this was a weird sentence to write, I'll be honest) and stifle my breathing. It's not something I've ever shared with people, but I did it a lot as a child. I took my dressing gown cord, locked myself in the bathroom and tightened it around my neck. (Oh Christ, now I'm panicking about the emergency escape rope I keep under my children's beds. What was I thinking?)

The sensation of not being able to breathe was so soothing and peaceful. (Do not try this at home. It is dangerous and you could die. These days I go for a run or take myself off somewhere quiet and take deep breaths. Far safer, and far less awkward to write about in a book.)

If being honest about how you feel is not something you have learned to do and if, like me, you live in fear of people being cross with you, then lying can become the only way to get out of doing something you don't want to do or going somewhere you don't want to be. 'Thank you for the opportunity, but this job isn't for me,' is a perfectly acceptable thing to say, but instead I'd go with 'My grandad has died. We were very close and I can't come in today.' And then, I'd never turn up again. My grandad has died about eight times. In reality, he died just once, long before I was born, which made faking his death less morally problematic (I think). As a grown woman, any situation which might require an honest expression of how I felt filled me with anxiety and was to be buried under lies.

'I am fond of you, but this relationship isn't working for me. I don't want to be romantically intimate with you anymore' is also an acceptable thing to say, yet 'I think I'm a lesbian' was easier for me when I wanted to get out of the short-lived relationships of my twenties.

I was a fairly prolific shoplifter in my twenties and old enough to get into serious trouble for it. I had come to accept this 'weird' part of me. It was my deep secret, before I understood there was something driving me to get these dopamine hits. I stole mainly sanitary products and make-up. In a huge supermarket, I once stole an eyeshadow. It beeped when I went past the till. (Who puts a security tag on a tiny Rimmel eyeshadow? Tight bastards!)

The woman at the till said, 'Have you got something in your pockets?'

'No!' I said and turned back to go into the aisles, my heart pounding. 'I've forgotten something!'

Do not leave the store. I knew that. They cannot do you for stealing from the store if you are still in it. I dashed about the aisles, making a pantomime of trying to look for something, completely aware that a security guard was now following me. By the deep freezers, I put my hand in my pocket, hid the eyeshadow in my fist, then reached deep down into the freezer. I dropped the eyeshadow in, picked up a pack of fish fingers, briefly examined it, then put it back and left the shop. Relief washed over me as I hotfooted it away from the store and I never went back, even though I lived around the corner. I should mention at this point that I didn't even wear eyeshadow back then.

A horror almost as bad as waking up with a stranger I did not remember bringing home, was waking up to find other people's belongings I had brought home. At least the strangers returned themselves. More than a few times, I had to retrace my steps and anonymously put on doorsteps items I had taken from house parties. These pilgrimages of shame and regret have seen me return a fancy umbrella, bottles of expensive shampoo and conditioner, and once, quite a large ornamental rhino which I had to return to a house in Dalston.

I never, ever planned to steal. Looking back, I shouldn't even have been at those parties. The noise, too many strangers – I never enjoyed them, and they were not situations I felt comfortable in so I drank and stole. The next day: 'HELLO, GUILT! Come in, sit down and bounce a cannonball on my chest!' As it pummelled my body, I imagined the person whose house we were at, looking forward to a lovely shower to wash away their hangover and the cigarette smoke in their hair, only to find some arsehole had nicked their shampoo. I was sure everyone would know it was me. *Who was that girl? The fat Asian one with frizzy hair? It was her, I'm sure it was her. She was such a weirdo.* These imaginary conversations people were having about me whirled round and round in my head. The ruminations would not leave me alone – *Nobody actually wants you at parties, they feel sorry for you, they are all cool and know you are not, they all hate you, they are all calling each other up today talking about how annoying you are.*

Shame is not to be confused with being embarrassed. When my swimming costume split in swim classes at school and my bum was exposed, I was embarrassed. When I stole from my classmates, lied and put Karen Keyworth's shoe in the loo, that was pure, painful, burning shame. As an adult, I simply found more things to feel ashamed of. Life got bigger and emotions more complicated, and navigating them with undiagnosed ADHD led to a whole tapestry of impulsive behaviours, doing a whole lot of damage and creating giant pits of shame upon shame upon shame. I know now that shame lurks inside your darkest corners, hidden away; but it breeds and gets bigger and darker and haunts your logical mind. Confronting shame is the only way to stop it eating you up; this is what therapy has taught me. When I did not understand my brain, how it worked, what it lacked, while I still thought there was something in *me* that was weird and wrong and broken, I was far from being able to control impulses which hurt me and other people, and was unable to confront my shame. It grew and caused me more and more problems as my ADHD remained undiscovered and untreated.

THE 'FUCK IT' BUTTON

In *Pretty Woman*, Richard Gere's character sits in a giant hot tub with Julia Roberts in her 'adorable sex worker' role and tells her it cost him thousands in therapy to say, 'I am very *angry* with my father.' Similarly, it cost me quite a lot of money in therapy to say, 'I'll think about it and get back to you.' What seems to come naturally to most people took me hours and hours of understanding my brain to be able to do.

Learning to say, 'Let me think about it', has changed my life for the better. A game changer. It buys time, so you can politely say no if you don't want to, say, look after someone's three dogs and iguana for a whole week. I no longer do things that sap my energy and eat my time, just to please other people. I don't mean I've become a complete arsehole and stopped doing favours for my friends and neighbours; I just don't take on what I cannot manage.

For example, here's a few things I've said 'yes!' to without considering the impact they'll have on me:

- 'Can a friend I met in India and knew for five days stay at your house with her four children for two weeks?'
- 'Can you come to the opening of my play a week after you have had a caesarean?'

- 'Do you mind if I dye my hair at your house because my flatmates hate the mess it makes in our bathroom?'
- 'Can you do this comedy/writing job for no money that will take up your entire day?'
- 'Can I keep my drugs at your flat and deal from there, because my girlfriend doesn't like me doing it from home?'
- 'A man I met in the pub last night who has just come out of prison needs a place to stay. Can he stay at yours?'

I agreed to all of these things and a zillion others, without allowing myself time to think through the consequences. The 'man just out of prison' came to live in the spare room of my ramshackle student accommodation, bringing a huge dog with him. I was a 20-year-old student and he was a bloke in his thirties, WHO HAD JUST COME OUT OF PRISON! (I didn't know what he'd been in for; I thought it rude to ask.) The dog shit everywhere and the man never paid the rent he promised he would and there was always a strange rustling coming from his room.

His room was next to mine and one day, when he was out, I went in to take a peek. The door was hard to open. I forced it and saw what was blocking the way: the entire floor was about 2 foot deep in newspaper. There was a path to his bed where he had waded through it. That night, he came in from the pub and screamed outside my room, 'I'M GOING TO KILL YOU!' Telling his dog, 'KILL THE STUDENT BITCH! KILL HER!' The poor, sweet doggie did not kill me, but I was freaked out regardless and rolled under the bed to hide. Yet IT DIDN'T OCCUR TO ME TO ASK ANYONE FOR HELP. I did not have any sense of boundaries or what was 'normal'. Was it fine to let a man move in with you whose surname you did not know, who brought his belongings round in a clear plastic bag with HM PRISON SERVICE on it and who threatened to set his dog on you at night? I had no clue.

Even the fact that I lived in a huge, dilapidated house that was in such disarray was evidence that looking after myself was not a priority. It had a couple of bathrooms, a creepy cellar, two kitchens and a hodgepodge of people living in it who never spoke to me. I have no idea why. Oh, it might have been because I invited a stranger with a shady history and an un-housebroken dog to live with us. Perhaps that was it.

My ADHD brain was very keen to, above all, please other people, without considering that while you are trying to please one person you could be really inconveniencing others. One afternoon part of the bathroom ceiling collapsed as I was laying in the bath. It was this and, bizarrely not the death threat, that was the last straw. I sat in the bath covered in plaster and masonry dust and thought, *It's time to go.*

I moved into a flat with two friends at university who enjoyed smoking weed. I did not. Both were forthright people and I found them quite intimidating (not being friends with people I found intimidating was another lesson I took my sweet time learning). They excitedly told me the local dealer was going to give us scraps in return for 'storing his gear at our flat and selling from here!' This did not seem like a good deal to me. If he was a baker and baked from our place and let us keep some cupcakes each time then yes, I was up for it. But now our flat was a place people trooped in and out of buying weed, smoking some with the dealer to make sure it was good stuff. I did not like it, so I told my intimidating flat-mates, 'This decision was made without asking me. I pay the same rent as you and so it's not fair. Plus, are you too stupid to realise that if he gets caught, it's us who will be in possession and not him?'

I am lying. Of course I didn't say this. Far too honest and scary. Sangeeta, a friend of mine who was visiting from Manchester, saw what was going on. She was not intimidated by anyone. 'They are taking the piss, Shap,' she said. 'Leave this to me.' It was she who made the dealer come round, take his gear and scarper, never to darken our door again. (Thanks, Sangeeta.)

My inability to speak my mind or stand up for myself for fear of risking an argument is something I must have learned at a very young age, while my parents fought or when my father was having one of his dark moods and our only prayer of avoiding his wrath was being utterly quiet and compliant. The absolute terror of people being disappointed or cross with me comes, I think (my therapist thinks), from my father's very up-and-down mood swings. ADHD has hereditary elements and, while I am not a psychiatrist and he has never been assessed, I am as sure as I can be that my father has ADHD too. He cannot sit still, unless he is writing. He has never seen a whole film through to the end. He is full of verve and excitement, which depletes and he naps suddenly, like a puppy, wherever he happens to be.

He also has 'the switch', the moment his temper flies because he has burned himself out, overloaded with stress, and has not processed his emotions. In my father, this manifested itself by him bellowing with his entire being at his small children for holding a fork incorrectly. If he had been able to take a moment and connect with himself, he would have understood that his anxiety was not fork-related. Even as a child, I could see my father's rages were separate from who he really was. That knowledge didn't help a bit, though, when my bones were rattling from his roars that went on and on until he had exhausted himself. He would, after a day or two, become 'wonderful Dad' again, and you could hold your fork any old way you wanted and he wouldn't care. Then, after a while, we would feel the tremors build up again and we would hold our breath, hold our forks carefully and correctly. But he would find something: a sock on the floor, an ill-judged wisecrack, and *BOOM!* 'Scary, rattle-your-bones Dad' would be back like a storm.

'Come for a pint!'

In the 1990s, binge-drinking culture was led by celebrity 'ladettes'. The ladette culture was young women muddling 'feminism' up with 'alcoholism'. 'He's drinking ten pints, why can't I?' Because, Shap, you are 5 foot 2 inches. You will die. In a way, it was a reaction to years of being objectified, taking the power back by railing against being ladylike. The ladettes behaved worse than the lads: 'I'm going to be sick on my dress and piss in the street – TAKE THAT, THE PATRIACHY!'

But, whatever the sociocultural reasons, there is no one this lifestyle lends itself to more than a massively insecure young woman with undiagnosed ADHD. I drank and drank and drank. When other girls stopped and started to build more adult lives, I did not. If you have ADHD, alcohol can be a way to slow down that motor. Without it, in a social situation, with noise and lots of people, I would literally feel things fizzing and popping inside me. My motor revved up wildly, unable to process new people, chat, noise, anxiety, excitement – it all whirled inside me, overwhelming me, and then booze – lovely, soothing booze – levelled me out, slowed my brain down, made me feel normal. But I couldn't stop until I was totally trollied.

At first, it would be confidence juice. There was no social anxiety in the 1990s – you were just 'paranoid'. I would promise myself, swear to myself, that I would have a glass of water for every pint, but could never stick to it. I never planned to get blotto. But I would, every time I went out. And I would go out every night.

The choices I made in these conditions were not great; none of the 'self-care' you hear about these days went on for me. Like going home with a stranger from the pub or club. There is nothing wrong with a one-night stand, if it's what you want and you are both on the same page. But I did not do it because I'd decided to have some carefree sexy fun. I did it because I had pressed the 'Fuck It' button.

The 'Fuck It' button is mostly a self-destruct button. You press it when you know you need to keep your wits about you but the pressure is too great and you decide to check out, responsibility-wise. Perhaps there is someone there you are in danger of bonking and really shouldn't, because you know it will make you feel bad, and you should go home to bed instead of staying out and boozing. Perhaps you have something important you want a clear head for – a 7am recording for *Celebrity Mastermind*, for example (I came last). Or maybe your grandmother is in hospital in a coma and you want to be there when she dies.

I got wasted and had a one-night stand when I should have been at my grandmother's bedside. It was 1997, I was 23, and I was eyeballs-deep in bulimia and binge-drinking. I had started to do some stand-up gigs but my main source of income was working in a call centre in Farringdon. The evening shift finished at 9pm and most nights – every night – a gang of us would tumble into the pub. This night, though, I needed to get to the hospital. But I was disconnected from my emotions. I didn't want to feel them; I only knew how to smother them.

I had visited my gran earlier in the day, before work, and stupidly thought she was coming out of her coma, even though we had been told there was no chance. She had squeezed my hand and sat up. I thought she was going to speak but she projectile-vomited blood and fell back down again. It is absolutely insane that I went into work after that. Can you imagine? I was completely unable to acknowledge what I actually needed, that I was *allowed* to have a break. *JUST KEEP GOING. NEVER STOP TO THINK.*

So at 9pm, when a good-looking courier who had just made a delivery got in the lift as I was leaving looked at me and said, 'Drink?' I said 'Yes!', because this was my default answer and I never thought about what the consequences would be.

It was horrible sex in a horrible flat in Barons Court, with horrible lipstick in the bathroom and other women's things, which indicated his girlfriend was away. The next morning, he showed none of the interest or friendliness of the night before. He didn't even want to hear about the time I met The Krankies. I shut his horrible front door and realised I'd left my nice jacket there. I had to ring the bell. He tossed it to me, out of the window, without a word. Horrible, stupid, awful night.

Full of hangover and self-loathing, I knew my gran had gone even before I got a call from my mum, as I was on the way to the tube.

Alcohol had become a problem long before this, though. I was 17 the first time I got black-out drunk. A boy from my school, who I shall call 'The Angel', liked me. He was talented and gorgeous, and nobody like him had fancied me before. He was shy and quiet and this party had been thrown, in true teenage style, so we could get together. I was shy too, so I drank vodka and orange juice from a jug until I was utterly wasted. The Angel had a car, was sober and took me home. I had no recollection of it. My friend, who also got a lift home, told me they had to stop the car twice for me to be sick. I woke up in my bed the next day to find I had wet myself.

I staggered into the bathroom to find puke across the wall. My grandmother lived with us at the time and was in a proper old huff with me. 'Please! Please talk to me,' I wept. I adored my gran. She was funny and we loved each other. I was horrified that my getting drunk had so appalled her.

But it wasn't just that. She told me, 'You were deranged last night. I got you a glass of water and you stood on your bed, yanked down your pants and pissed yourself. *Then …*' she added indignantly, 'you told me to "eat shit". But now you feel like shit, so that is your punishment. Now go and get clean and I will give you a cuddle.'

My mother thought the drinking was because I was in a 'bad crowd'. I really wasn't. My friends were still the geeks and the nerds. Nobody else had got into the state I had. My mother is teetotal and very straight-laced (unlike my father, who is a monkey). She was very strict about me going out as a teenager: 'You are not staying the night at Caroline's house! I do not want you to end up like Michelle on *Eastenders*.' (In case you do not have forensic knowledge of 1980s *Eastenders* like me, Michelle Fowler got pregnant by her best mate Sharon's dad, Dennis Watts, during a sleepover at Sharon's house.) Caroline was my friend from school who was a devout Catholic and was genuinely considering becoming a nun. I was only 14 and mortified my mother would imagine such a thing. I was nowhere near as pretty as Michelle Fowler. There was no way a friend's predatory middle-aged dad would ever fancy me!

My father was a boozer, a highly functioning one. He is a bohemian type and a poet and understood my need for hedonism and freedom but didn't, in those days, connect binge-drinking with something deeper that needed to be addressed. 'Just stop when you are still having a good time,' was his attitude. I couldn't. I couldn't 'just' anything.

The ladettes have grown up now; the generation gap between us and our children is smaller. We know the signs to look out for, we know the damage to your mental health drinking to excess will inflict. A few years ago, my friend's teenage daughter got black-out drunk on a school trip. She was 17. My friend took her daughter to AA meetings for teenagers where she got to be in a room and actually talk about her feelings with people who were also sharing theirs. A year or two later, she was diagnosed with ADHD. She got some extra help with her studying and continues to go to AA meetings, where she can connect with her peers on a meaningful level. WOW. How incredible that this can be what happens now. It's useless to wish I had had that kind of support – however chaotic I was, every path my life took me down has led to my son and daughter, my dogs and cats and living within walking distance of at least four exquisitely friendly coffee shops. That said, I am in awe of my friend and how far we have come with looking after struggling young people and recognising self-medication.

I love the way young people now talk about self-care. When I was in my twenties, 'self-care' was having a glass of water before bed and a proper rummage around yourself on a Sunday morning to check you hadn't left a condom up there.

Thankfully, our culture has changed. My teenage son will say 'no thanks' to a friend's invite to go out if he has already had a busy week and needs to chill. I was not like this as a young person. I suffered over the invites I *wasn't* getting and would move heaven and earth to get to the ones I *was*, never stopping to consider that sometimes, I did not even want to go.

When I was in my teens and twenties, there was a general acceptance that getting shit-faced was a rite of passage every young person goes through. So many of us who were self-medicating went unchecked. *YOU* were the problem, not the world you couldn't fit into, the systems that didn't serve you, the pressures you couldn't talk about. At university, the freedom of being able to go out as late as I wanted without permission was dizzying. At home every party I went to, every night out, had to be explained to my mother. Her permission depended on how relentless my reassurance was and how persistent my begging. Understandable, I suppose, after the 'eat shit, grandma' incident and the shenanigans of people on *Eastenders*.

At university, the excitement of so many new people and being *free* was off the scale. We were all in the same boat – away from home and out to make friends and have as much fun as possible. Alcohol seemed to be what it was all about and on the first night, in the student union, I got drunk, very drunk, and found myself snogging a guy who I did not fancy at all, in full view of all these new people who I'd be spending the next three years around. Mortifying. I was a virgin who had only ever kissed three people, and each had been a huge deal. Now here I was with the tongue of a boy from 'the West Country' (where was *that*?) in my mouth. 'Are you going home with Shappi?' someone asked him. What? People did that? Did people think I would do that? I had zero experience in this sort of thing. Also, my mother would be so ashamed. 'No way!' I said and ran out, followed by a girl I had made friends with, who walked me back to my student accommodation where I shared a bedroom with a girl from Tunbridge Wells who had stayed in to organise her side of the room. (She was a quiet type who liked Jammie Dodgers. The following term, my friend Jane swapped rooms with her and shared with me instead. We had more in common, like staying out late and being sick on our beds. Jane and I remain firm friends to this day.)

Despire the Ladette culture of 'blokes do it, why can't we?', the term 'slag' was a label both men and women slapped on those who got off with guys when they were shit-faced. 'Sex positive' was a concept decades away for the likes of me. I was regularly crushed with shame after a night out, where a stranger's tongue had found its way into my mouth. *SHAME, SHAME! SHE'S A SLAG!*, I imagined people thought. When you are locked into a booze-fuelled ADHD paranoia, it's hard to remember that most people are wrapped up in their own lives and rarely give a second thought to what you're up to.

Many people at university, it turned out, were sexually active, like it was normal. Sex! A few of my friends in London had sex and I lived in fear of my mother finding out *they* were doing it, let alone considering doing it myself. It was unthinkable. *What would my mother say?* I thought in horror. *Why would she be watching?* didn't cross my mind. It didn't matter if she wasn't actually there; it would feel like she was. She wouldn't let me steal a few strawberries; she wasn't going to be happy about me having a penis inside me. See how irrational shame is? It's illogical, but all-powerful.

There was no way I was going to have any sex. My mother being there in spirit aside, I would have to actually get naked with a boy, speak to him and probably have some eye contact, and I did not know how to do things like that. All the friends I made at university were girls. Partly because there were 12 women to every 3 guys at King Alfred's College. Remarkably, I did not see a problem with this when I applied. Another reason was because my experience of boys so far had been that they teased me and filled me with stress, so I was terrified of them. I became a 'fag hag', a term that has not withstood the test of time, but meaning a girl whose only male friends were homosexual. My mother was absolutely fine with LGBTQ friends because they tended to hug her a lot and were unlikely to get me pregnant.

People attribute my mother's attitude around me and sex to the fact that she is Iranian; that it was a cultural thing. But I met my gran, my mother's mother, when I was about 12 and she was finally able to visit from Iran. My gran was very open-minded and told filthy jokes with a sparkle in her eye, to my mother's horror.

'Slag' and 'slut' were still normal words to throw at girls. I was friends with young feminists who railed against the terms but they were in a minority and branded 'militants'. We had Germaine Greer and *The Female Eunuch*, but I really could have done with Cardi B and Lizzo. Before you say, 'But you had Madonna!' No, I didn't. Madonna was too cool. Madonna had been little help to girls like me, who were quieter types. Lizzo is a geek. She plays the flute, for goodness' sake. Thank God for flute-playing, geeky, sex-positive role models, who, like me, are also not white. A rarity in the mainstream.

Until I went to university, I had no idea that not being an Anglo-Saxon was of note to anyone other than the National Front. Now, boys would either tell me, 'I fancy Asian birds' or 'You're alright but I don't go for Asian birds.' The need to let you know whether or not they wanted to bonk you was very prevalent amongst the 'laddy' lads. The girls brought it up too. Mostly with the well-meaning, 'You're so lucky you have a natural tan!' One girl from the Isle of Wight asked me if I was circumcised. It was no wonder that the small cluster of Londoners at my college gathered together. The one Black guy I knew at college, the one Asian guy, a Jewish guy, a Black girl and my roommate, Jane, all clung on to each other in that first term.

I remained a virgin until my third year at university. I did 'everything but'. 'Everything but' got me thrown out of a pub, a nightclub and involved many other mortifying, unsatisfying drunken encounters.

When I moved back home after university, I carried on drinking, shouting at my parents, 'EVERYONE DOES IT!' when they worried about me. My father tried to be understanding: 'Drink alcohol, but don't let the alcohol eat you.'

Pithy little sayings don't really work when you have a raging booze problem.

What nobody realised, including myself, was that I was in a constant state of anxiety and alcohol gave me respite from it. It weirdly quietened down my ADHD brain at first, but then I couldn't stop and would regularly black out.

My first novel, *Nina is Not OK*, is about a teenage alcoholic. I lied to every journalist who asked if any of it was autobiographical. Of course it was. Not all of it, but much of it was lifted from my life at university, and the decade after it, when I sank into booze.

'You get to a point with wine that you are not *you* anymore,' my close friend told me after she had had to peel me off the floor and take me home from a party. 'You were looking at me last night but you weren't there.' But how did you stop? How did anyone stop? How were other people able to go home before they had to be carried?

Once I started stand-up comedy and gigging regularly, there was plenty of opportunity to booze with other comedians after shows. I ran around like I had a firework up my bum at parties, comedy clubs and pubs. Because I was shy. And alcohol gave me the confidence to feel like I was part of what was going on and not deal with any of the anxiety around this high-risk career choice. ADHD does not care about your mental health. It never ushers you home early to put a mug of Horlicks in your hand. For me, there was only ever one choice: press the 'Fuck It' button, leap into booze, pretend you are having a good time then binge your way through your hangover.

My life was filled with mayhem and the far-from-ideal situations I ended up in. It was normal, back then, when we couldn't afford taxis, to kip at the house of another comedian, who lived nearby. I was at a club in south-east London, very far from my home in Ealing, west London, and a comic I had just met offered me a bed for the night. He was the compère and I was doing an open spot, so as far as I was concerned, he was Tom Cruise and I was a fledgling actor trying to get a break. My comic friend Patrick Monahan had already said I could stay at his. I felt safe with him. But when this other comic offered, a bloke I had met THAT NIGHT – 'I'm only around the corner, easier to stay at mine' – I said yes, because he was Tom Cruise and I didn't want him to think I was rude. Patrick said, 'Are you sure, mate?' But the other comic was standing with us and I didn't want him to feel awkward. Did my feminist sisters at the back all hear that? I WENT HOME WITH A STRANGE MAN BECAUSE I DID NOT WANT TO MAKE HIM FEEL AWKWARD.

I had every right to change my mind. However, my brain was immobilised. I was unable to take a breath, take a step back and make a decision that incorporated a degree of self-care.

So I stayed at the stranger's house and he did indeed make sexual advances towards me. (By that I mean he took out his guitar and sang to me. In the 1990s, this was one move away from getting your cock out. In most cases, it was worse.) When

I told him I did not wish to copulate with him, he left and went to a party. Oh, and before he left, he said, 'I'm gonna get in bed with you when I get back' and locked me in his flat.

I waited until he was gone a few minutes, then assessed how many bones I would break if I jumped out of the window. Too many, I decided. I was on the second floor. There was a Turkish restaurant across the road. 'EXCUSE ME!', I shouted to waiters closing up. They ran to help. A ladder was fetched, a strong Turkish man climbed up to help, his arms not quite reaching the window. I climbed out anyway and he grabbed my legs to help me down. The restaurant owner paid for my cab home.

This should not have been the end of an evening of *work*, while I was trying to make my stand-up routine a career. It wasn't a one-off. I don't mean I was regularly re-enacting *Rapunzel* to escape potential sexual assault. I mean I was drinking too much to mask the anxiety and attempt to quiet my ever-whirring brain, which was constantly galloping away at top speed, making terrible decisions, while I hung on for dear life. None of which was good for my well-being or my career. The worst was when unwanted, unasked-for sex happened.

There was one time, when I was out late after a gig, had no money for a cab home and a guy persuaded me I was safer staying at his house than if I got on the night bus. If I had the awareness I do now, I would have gone straight to the police and reported that I had been assaulted. The #MeToo movement was hard for me initially. In the 1990s, we young women would take pride in seeming bulletproof, being boozy and wild. At the time, I was trying to make it in an industry that was male-dominated and it was rare to see two women billed together. I didn't want to make a fuss. And to whom would I have even made a fuss? I did not want to face what had happened to me; it was all buried deep and I told myself 'regret is not rape!' But I had said, even before we got to his house, 'I don't want to have sex. Can you stay on the sofa?'. 'Yes', he assured me, but didn't I lay there thinking, 'This is his house, what if he gets angry if I scream?' Yes. I definitely would have gone to the police if this happened now. But back then, in the putrid quicksand of shame, I blamed myself. We use the term 'the walk of shame' so casually, like it's a joke. It's not funny. No sexual encounter should carry this crushing, destructive stigma.

The first female comedian I made friends with was from Canada. We went out after a gig, and at the pub, she asked the barman for a tea. I said, 'A tea? A fucking tea? No, no, no, you are NOT having a tea; if you have a fucking tea you are *not* hanging out with us. Your career in this country is over. HAHAHA. TEA!'

She sat away from my table with some lovely, nerdy comedians because I was being an obnoxious twat. Truth was, I envied them. I envied the comics who stayed sober, or just not wasted, and talked about comedy and music and had a laugh. I could not be calm enough to do that, to listen to people in a group, to sit my arse down on a chair when there was so much else going on around me.

A friend of mine, an American girl I met in Germany, declared at 18 that she was an alcoholic and has never touched booze since. Her 'rock bottom' was that she went out and drank so much that she woke up at a stranger's house without having a clue how she got there. That was a fairly standard weekly occurrence for me. Rather than consider she was right, that drinking yourself unconscious is a sign that you have a drink problem, I took the piss out of her to all my friends. 'Hahaha! She thinks she's an alcoholic but I do that ALL THE TIME. AH HA HA!'

Most people who drink are familiar with The Horrors the next day when you have a hangover. 'Oh God! What did I say? Why did I do that?' With ADHD, emotional dysregulation and hypersensitivity make The Horrors go nuclear. The morning after I'd been drunk, my very existence was a calamity. If I was to switch on the TV, a news reporter would surely say, 'The whole country, and indeed the entire world, had its eyes opened yesterday to what a disgraceful human being Shappi Khorsandi is. It has been confirmed that nobody at all likes her. She is annoying. Groups of cool people all over the world are hanging out together, drinking tea, having a great time and all agreeing that she is just about the worst person.'

I did not know that science played a part in how I was feeling, that for someone with ADHD, neurons are deficient in dopamine transporters. I had no idea, on all those booze binges, through all those demonic hangovers, that I was literally chasing dopamine. When we were together, my ex-husband would get exasperated by how much I drank. 'It was lunch with my family. Why are you in this state?', he would ask as he brought me home early. I never planned it. I just poured it down me like I was putting out a fire. One year, at the Melbourne International Comedy Festival, I met up with an old friend, Sally, from my university days. Sally was great fun and the two of us would get drunk and run up on the canteen roof, which started as a low slope then went up to about 30 feet. Stupid and dangerous of us. I shudder still when I remember us peering over the edge, off our faces. On a night out in Melbourne, I noticed Sally wasn't drinking. She told me she was a recovering alcoholic and hadn't drunk since she was 25. 'Don't you remember what I was like? I'd get black-out drunk! I never knew when or how to stop.' I was the same, exactly the same as her, but I could not stop.

That year in Melbourne, I was in the catastrophic storm of my marriage break-up. My son had been with me for the first part of the festival but then a relative of mine had come to take him back to London, to his dad. I couldn't bear being separated from my son for so long. I'd had choices, I could have insisted he stay with me, but I hadn't wanted even more friction between me and his dad, so I paid for my aunt to fly out with us and take him home, completely underestimating how I would feel about my son being in a different hemi-sphere to me. I threw myself into an ocean of beer.

I drank so much that another comedian sat me down and told me he thought I had a drink problem. The lifestyle of comedians is not known to be the healthiest, especially in my generation. The 4am bedtimes, 2am service station dinners and the general lack of respect for your liver. So when another comic tells you you're drinking too much, it is like a priest telling you to 'ease up on the God stuff'. But I couldn't stop, even though I was getting night sweats because my liver was sobbing and wailing under its workload.

I'm not putting the blame for all this purely at the door of ADHD. I wish I could. It's far easier than to accept there were huge vaults inside me, inside my emotional storage, boxes crammed with STUFF I had not dealt with. Like with most human beings, there had been painful episodes in my life and I had left the emotions around them to fester. If I had known I had ADHD, would I have waded through all these and sorted them out sooner? Who knows. I cannot say. I do know that the lower your self-esteem, the less likely you are to confront your anxiety, to be able to imagine it as something separate from you, something you can manage or even banish.

The science around this isn't definite, but it could be that trauma can exacerbate ADHD symptoms, which is why the notion that medication as the first port of call is problematic. Even if I had been given ADHD medication much earlier in my life, the pills themselves would not have helped me to process the catastrophic aftermath of the 1979 Iranian Revolution, which had catapulted my family and me into exile. (Although they may have helped me pack more efficiently.) If I had been diagnosed at 15 and given pills to deal with what I was experiencing, would that really have helped me in the long run? Or would it, back in 1988, have made me feel that I was 'mad' and cause me to reject help because of the stigma?

Medication, in my case an amphetamine, is nothing without a scaffolding of support from humans and nature. Therapy, meditation, fresh air and the feel of grass under your feet quieten down your motor and are key to managing ADHD, at least in my experience. The first thing that happened, when I started to realise I had ADHD in my forties and began to see a therapist, was that my anxiety subsided. Until that happened, I didn't even know it was there. Identifying this feeling I'd always lived with and, crucially, learning that I could actually do something about it was like discovering a fake wall in your house and finding out that you could move it, revealing a beautiful new house that was much nicer, brighter and tidier than the one you'd been living in. I hadn't known that the raging feelings of paranoia and anxiety could be moved. No wonder I drank; no wonder I used booze and food and sex to give myself temporary respite from the debilitating anxiety in my head and in my guts. You have to learn what anxiety is before you realise you have it, otherwise you don't even know you have it. After all, 'a dog doesn't know it's a dog'. (I wish this was a quote from Confucius, but no, I heard it on The Chris Evan's Radio Show'.)

I am writing this chapter on 3 January 2023. I had a karaoke party on New Year's Eve and I did not drink. A combination of ADHD medication and the perimenopause mean my tolerance towards alcohol has significantly lowered. Just one glass of wine feels like I've had ten coffees and robs me of sleep, so hangovers are off-the-scale horrific.

On New Year's Eve, I knew I did not want to feel wretched the next day. ADHD management helps me to consider consequences and act accordingly. This might sound so normal to some people, as though I am saying, 'I learned that if I stick my hand into a fire, it will hurt, so I no longer do that.' But if you have ADHD, you will understand that it's something to *know* what's best for you and something quite different to be able to act on it.

I was actually able to think, *Do I want New Year's day to be a hellish write-off? No, so I shall not drink.* So at the little party I had on New Year's Eve, while my friends drank, I had alcohol-free lager. At midnight, instead of the pink champagne, I mixed Ribena and fizzy water then sang, 'I Will Survive' on karaoke. I had fun. Yes. But my friends undoubtedly had more fun. I soberly watched them beautifully murder classics. I watched them howl with laughter and misbehave. I was reminded that I am not naturally gregarious. I am quite quiet. But I knew I would not wake up with a head full of self-hate; my children would not watch me drag myself through the next day. I would not have to talk my anxiety down to a manageable size. I watched my mate sing Chas & Dave's 'Ain't No Pleasing You' as though he was on stage at Madison Square Garden and thought, *How wonderful you are having so much fun* and then *Would it be rude if I left my guests to it and went to bed?*

THE IMPOSSIBLE THING

This is the chapter I have been dreading. Let's get on with it. My name's Shaparak Khorsandi and I am a compulsive over-eater and bulimic.

Of all the addictions, bulimia has had the least cinematic success. Al Pacino's Scarface would not have become an iconic character if, in the final scene, instead of a mountain of cocaine, Tony Montana had stuck his head in a Tesco's Finest baked Alaska. Alcohol has *Leaving Las Vegas*, heroin has *Trainspotting*, but no compelling, cinematic darkness can be brought to a scene where someone is locked in a bathroom, crouching by the loo, desperately trying to yak out all of their Sunday dinner while family or friends knock on the door, wondering why they have been in there for half an hour.

In the artistic world, some addictions are almost roman-ticised. Hemingway and William S. Burroughs were both addicts, for example. Neither of these facts diminished people's regard for them; far from it. To this day, people go to Jim Morrison's grave and leave bottles of booze and joints. Elton John had bulimia. Thankfully, he recovered. If he hadn't, though, I doubt fans, if he had left us, would embark on pilgrimages to leave Pringles and a Colin the Caterpillar cake at his shrine.

Unless you look under the bed and find all the hidden wrappers and empty boxes of Mr Kipling, bulimia is hard to spot. Eating is what everyone does, so you can abuse your substance in plain sight. Five helpings of treacle pudding at a wedding buffet is easier to get away with than firing up a crack pipe during the speeches.

From early childhood, I had a compulsion to eat and keep eating. I have a memory of being at nursery and having anxiety because if, at juice and biscuit time, I did not get to sit right by the plate of biscuits, thus increasing my chances of getting two, I would definitely combust. For my Iranian family, dinners are banquets; no one keeps an eye on how much you eat. I would eat until I physically couldn't eat any more. Or breathe. Or move much. I became fat. Not massively fat, just fat enough to be shamed for it by the adults around me. 'You greedy little piggy!', they would say and pinch my belly, because I grew up in the days where adults were bloody idiots.

Other teenagers around me were enjoying drugs, but drugs terrified me. People told me about acid trips they had: 'I walked along the road, then it turned into a river, so I walked over it really slowly, trying not to fall in. And when I went home, my mum was Bungle from *Rainbow* and she melted every time I laughed.' No thank you. Acid was not for me.

I once got high on skunk and as my friend was talking to me, really intently, her head turned into a perfect triangle. A giant triangle that kept talking. *Fuck that*, I thought. *Drugs are not for me.* I did enjoy Es for a while. I loved them, in fact, but the downers when the weekend was over became horrific and I stopped with no fuss. Amphetamines were my drug of choice because they calmed me down. The way they work on an ADHD brain is different to a typical brain. They wake up the part that can organise the rest and so can quieten down the motor. So while everyone else took whizz to get high, I took it because it made me feel normal, focused.

Thinking about food, eating it and then throwing it back up dominated my life. I did this regularly when I was 16, obsessively at 18 and throughout my twenties, in some periods all day, for days and days and weeks on end. It started because I thought it would be a way to lose weight. I had seen a documentary about Elton John, who said he threw up food, and I thought, *What a marvellous idea!* The message I had got all my life was that I was too fat and greedy. From when I was very young, friends of my parents, random older Iranians I met at parties, took it upon themselves to tell me I was fat or chubby or, 'Honestly, Shaparak *jaan*, lose some weight and you'll see how pretty you actually are.' The prevailing culture of the time didn't help. In the 1990s, the fashion industry was accused of 'glamourising' anorexia by only using models who were extremely thin, sending out a message that if you could not wear a Polo mint as a garter you were a big fat hippo who should stay indoors because you were blocking out the sun. On top of that were comments from boys at school; being called 'the Incredible Bulk' and all the other playground nonsense as they tried to deal with their own insecurities by creating some for me.

'Urrgh! Look at the way she's eating her Mars bar!' boys said in my direction, in the canteen one day in secondary school as I sat, minding my own business. I was nibbling all the sides of the Mars bar, then the caramel, leaving the nougat till last (the *only* way to eat a Mars bar). '*Urghghgh*! Look at her! URGHGHGH!' The ring leader looked at me in disgust, forcing his mates to look at, and form an opinion on, my eating habits, and to agree I was disgusting.

'Yeah. AND she's fat,' offered one, limply. I had never had this kind of thing at primary school. Sure, people had called me fat and greedy but only adults, not *kids*. It pulled the rug right out from under me. I would have stood up for myself, said something cutting back, but my nervous system could not handle that. Best to bow my head and bottle it up, and convert it to self-hate. Much less risky than a confrontation.

In my teenage years, girls made out they didn't have an appetite because they thought it made them seem sexier. I found eating in front of boys excruciating. *Oh God, he's going to find out my body needs food to sustain it. He's probably thinking,* What a massive fat, greedy cow, needing to have *lunch*.

I wonder if the boys had a clue that was going on for us? I doubt it. I doubt any went home to ask their mum, 'Did you eat food when you were my age?'

I couldn't stop eating. I obsessed about food, then panicked I'd get fatter and so made myself puke. Compulsively eating a huge amount of food and then throwing it back up is not, in the end, about being thin because, to state the obvious, bulimia doesn't 'work'. There is no way you can expel all the calories of a binge. This is the biggest misconception about bulimia, that you eat some cake and throw it up because you don't want to get fat and then just get on with your day. Weight loss doesn't work like that. A binge might be one cake or one biscuit to one person, but it will be three packets of biscuits and a bag of doughnuts and four rounds of toast for another. You can't possibly get all of those calories out. That reality, though, did not stop me doing it. I began to eat and make myself sick regularly. I kept going because I discovered that bingeing and purging gave me a moment's respite from that ADHD-powered motor that was constantly whirring in my head.

Bulimia made the simple phrase 'let's go out for a meal!' an invitation to hell. What? Sit at a table, with other people? And not be able to eat their food too? What if they have more chips than me? What if someone leaves half of their pudding? And they're too far away for me to ask to have it? To sit at a table in a restaurant and eat publicly, to not be able to eat food off other people's plates, can be agony for a bulimic. Also, you need to go to the loo and throw it up, and most restaurants haven't thought to have single, soundproof booths where you can chuck up your expensive meal without someone who's reapplying their lipstick hearing you. Covering up bulimia is grotty. Chocolate mousse foams and floats and is so hard to flush, and a big clue as to what you've been doing is by saying you have diarrhoea if somebody asks what's wrong. The effort you must go to, to hide what you are doing, is immense. It drained my energy, wiped me out, yet still didn't sate me.

Even with bloodshot eyes and a red raw throat I might say, 'You not finishing your chips? Yeah, I'll have them.'

I have panicked when I haven't found a place to throw up. I would buy chocolates and crisps after a night out, eat them all methodically on the train home, then be unable to bear it all inside me, digesting on the ten-minute walk back to my house. So I'd go into the park, late at night, and hurl behind a bush. Grim. Sorry to put you through reading this.

Bulimia is a compulsion, an addiction, which takes a hold of your life and immobilises you, just as drugs and alcohol can. It is not about being 'greedy' or having your cake and eating it (then throwing it up). When you are an addict, your compulsions are normal to you. So normal that it was only occasionally I considered that there were people who ate food and stopped when they were full and got on with doing other things. I didn't understand when people said, 'I'm not all that hungry; shall we get something and share it?' What? Are you insane? If I only have half what is put in front of me, I will die.

I didn't make the connection between how much I ate and throwing up. This is hard to explain to non-addicts, but while I knew the throwing up was painful and hard, I believed it had to be done to 'undo' the eating. I hadn't yet understood that the eating itself was driven by a need to fix something, to self-medicate. I might experience a few seconds of euphoria as I emptied my stomach and felt the mountain of food erupt out of me, but then I was engulfed in a fog of shame, self-loathing and sweaty, bloodshot regret as I cleaned up splashes on the loo seat, on the floor, on my clothes, when everything became about no one else finding out. The vomiting made me cloudy, dizzy; often I'd physically hurt. My throat would be sore, my stomach cramped. I felt heavier, not lighter. I worried: what if give myself a heart attack? What if I've given myself a stomach ulcer?

The knowledge and support I have now with ADHD helped me navigate the anxiety I felt around social situations, getting work done and dealing with admin. When I did not know, eating and purging briefly stifled that anxiety and so, despite the regret, the shame, the pain and worry that followed, I would, to my horror, do it again. Soon. Often, immediately after I was sick, I would do it over and over again, each time feeling worse until I was just too exhausted to carry on or I ran out of food. I was locked in a cycle of bulimia – this huge, hideous monster that kept me in chains and robbed me of so much happiness, health and tooth enamel.

My twenties were a blur of boozing, bingeing and the late nights of the comedy circuits while trying to forge a career in stand-up. I would get sporadic gigs, then nothing for weeks. What I did get wasn't paid; I had cleaning jobs and life modelling jobs to make ends meet. But I did have incredible support in the form of a very grown-up friend called Sally who had a nine-to-five job and her own flat, in which she invited me to live with her, rent free.

What an opportunity! Imagine! I could write jokes all day and put in the hours calling up comedy clubs, filling my diary, getting better so I'd get paid gigs and my dreams would come true. In my BAFTA acceptance speech I would thank Sally for her generosity and for giving me the artistic space I needed.

Except it didn't quite work out like that. In the four years that I lived with her, I didn't do much other than the same ten-minute routine in comedy clubs. My career did not move forward at all. I didn't seem to be able to wade through the sludge I was in. Sally would leave for work and I would promise her, and myself, that I would spend the day writing jokes and phoning comedy clubs, trying to get gigs. But I did not. I'd ring a comedy club and if they picked up, I'd panic and say, 'Wrong number!' then hate myself for being so utterly inept.

I sat in the flat in a cycle of eating and throwing up. Locked in a fog of food. The flat would be a mess when she got back. I couldn't tidy. I'd pick up something to put away, a tub of Philadelphia for example, wander around the flat, then leave it on the sofa. 'When I leave the house, do you just sit here and throw things around?' Amy asked me, smiling in that 'I have to pretend I find this funny but really it's fucking annoying' way. Food went missing and when Amy noticed, I would have to lie.

'You lent a box of Crunchy Nut to the neighbour?' she once asked.

'Yeah,' I said. 'She's a nurse on shifts and she'd run out of food for breakfast.'

'You're too friendly with people,' she said, shaking her head and adding *cornflakes* to her shopping list. Thankfully, Sally wasn't the 'get to know your neighbours' type of person. I was. I knew everybody in our block. She lived in that flat for years and now I was telling her she was surrounded by people who endlessly had an emergency need for random groceries. I made up stories about the Philadelphia having ants in it; a Muslim neighbour wanting to try bacon for the first time … I had all sorts of stupid stories about why food went missing. Again, telling utterly unnecessary lies, saying anything out of shame and terror of a potential emotional repercussion. Sally hadn't believed any of them, she told me years later. 'I know,' I said. 'That's what it's like with an addict. They lie, you know they are lying, they know you know, but you both know that acknowledging this will not help.'

I didn't really question what I was doing. It was a secret but very routine part of my existence. Like being a werewolf. There is a scene in *An American Werewolf in London* where the nice handsome American student is bouncing around his nurse girlfriend's flat. He is happy. He is excitable. He is on a high. When she leaves, he sits in her flat with ants in his pants. He can't settle. He goes to the fridge, tries to read, tries to watch TV; but he can't focus, can't settle. Then the horror starts. He can feel himself changing. He is conscious of it; it's terrifying but he can't stop it. He watches his hands elongate, hair sprout out and then the werewolf totally takes over. He is a monster with no access to the rational part of him which would make the decision *not* to run out into the night and rip people apart. He wakes up in a zoo, in the wolf enclosure, with no recollection of how he got there. I related to that scene for so long without realising why.

❁

In my mid-twenties, I went to Los Angeles for a few months with my brother, into the bosom of the large Iranian community there. We did a weekly stand-up night, packing out a little comedy theatre with an exclusively Iranian American audience (the second biggest immigrant community in LA is Iranian). We made new friends and stayed in some fabulous places belonging to my father's friends. I was derailed by the abundance of food in America. Obscenely large portions of the most fat-laden, gloopy, gooey, delicious food were on offer for next to nothing. Pizzas the size of tables, giant plates of hot cookie dough smothered in ice cream. But in LA, at the same time, there is the absolute insistence that everyone is as thin and ironed out as possible. How can they expect both?! I put on weight and yet my bingeing was off the scale. My puking could not keep up with my eating. My brief time in LA gave me space for a bit of reinvention; I was something of a novelty, being British Iranian and being a comic. I didn't feel like the dork I felt at home. It felt good, to not feel like a dork. I met a pianist called Ashkan who took me on an American-style date (no alcohol and no touching). He said, 'I really like you, but you are so disconnected from yourself. Your head is like two inches away from your neck.' He saw that something was wrong and had the care and confidence to try and talk to me about it. In response to his compassion, I took the piss. I did impressions of him to everyone, laughed at him and didn't see him much after that. I was floored that someone who I had been partying with had looked more closely and had seen there was something wrong. I was not ready to see it. I was very committedly masking, hiding the fact that I was locked away in this other, horrible world. Forgive me for sounding pretty LA here, but his was the first hand that reached out to me, wanting to help. I laughed and slapped it away.

I'm staying in my twenties for a bit longer. I had a tight band of friends in my twenties, made up of three sets of siblings and their close friends and partners. The majority of my gang were Iranians, raised in the UK like me. At Christmas, we made up for being first-generation Iranians who did not have traditional Christmases when we were growing up, because our parents had made saffron-infused turkey and served it with basmati rice. So one year, we gathered together at the house of Sammy and Cyrus's parents, which was large and fancy, and we had the most picture-perfect Christmas. We had carols, Secret Santa and turkey, goose and pheasant roasted to perfection, along with a nut roast for the vegetarian among us who, back in the 1990s, we regarded as some kind of shaman because she did not eat meat. There were mountains of roast potatoes and parsnips and every side dish you can think of, displayed on the most beautifully decorated table. Chocolate and cake were everywhere, and mince pies were served with ice cream. I pulled it all into my mouth, ploughing for hours.

I was in the toilet for the fourth time that Christmas Day, stretching out my foot to block the door in case someone tried to come in (fancy house, no lock on the door, baffling) and saw me leaning over the toilet, making myself sick. The operation took a considerable amount of dexterity and I felt lucky that I was so bendy. I'd eaten the chocolate after my dinner, so you'd think the endless lumps of Chocolate Orange and countless After Eights would have come out first, but I'd had to wait for someone else to come out of the loo and now puking was difficult. My stomach muscles ached as I forced them to churn up more food. More bloody parsnips, peas, carrots, all the good stuff was coming out, then, finally, mint! Hallelujah! The sickly sweetness of chocolate blended with the eye-watering bitterness of vomit found its way to my throat.

The angle of my leg by the door forced me to twist my body slightly over the loo seat so my stomach cramps were worse. I powered through, a trooper, forcing more of the chocolate out. My head began to hurt from the straining; my throat was sore. There was a full-length mirror to the side of the loo and, from my contorted angle, I suddenly caught sight of myself: eyes bloodshot, face blotchy and damp, finger in my mouth right down to the last knuckle. For the first time, the very clear thought rang in my head: *Oh. This isn't normal.*

I mean, I knew it wasn't normal, that's why I hid it from people, but I had been in this mindset that it was normal to *me*. It was more that other people wouldn't understand it. I hid it the way werewolves hide their true selves. If people knew, there would be a fuss. There had been people I had confided in along the way, never telling them the full extent of it, and they would say, 'Oh, but you're not fat!' Or 'God, you know you can die from that? You can burn a hole in your oesophagus and bleed to death.' Or 'That's so wasteful! Just stop!' None of this helped. None of it stopped me.

On that particular Christmas Day, for the first time, I properly understood that this hiding away, this secret gorging and puking was external to me, not part of who I was. That it wasn't like epilepsy or being allergic to eggs. It didn't occur to me until that moment that doing it in the first place was the problem, not people finding out. But how do you begin to explain to people your life is ruled by obsessive thoughts that lead to you repeatedly doing something so violent and damaging to your body? I had been doing this for so long that trying to explain to a therapist, or anyone else, what it was like from scratch was so hard, like telling people 'did you know I am really Superman?'. Years later, I did begin to ask for help. I went to my GP. Nothing much happened. I got put on a waiting list, then started to see a therapist who seemed very nice but didn't understand. When I made a little joke she said, unsmiling, 'You seem to use humour to mask your real feelings,' then jotted something down in her notebook.

'I hope you're writing down my joke. It was gold.'

She looked up briefly and said flatly, 'No. I am not.'

Dammit. I was dying on my arse in a therapy session. She asked me some questions about my family, then about my eating rituals. As I answered she kept looking up at the big clock on the wall behind me. Whenever she looked at the clock, that familiar feeling of being a nuisance and a hindrance to people crept through me, muttering, *See? SEE?*

Even your therapist doesn't like you. You are boring and your face isn't nice to look at.

'Let's get a food plan together for you,' the therapist said eventually. 'Stick to the meals we plan for each week and really stick to them.'

My problem wasn't that I didn't know to eat three meals a day. I wasn't accidentally eating too much. It wasn't as if I had forgotten I was meant to have just a bowl of porridge for breakfast then absent-mindedly ate an entire giant airport Toblerone. It was like telling an alcoholic, 'Instead of having three bottles of wine at breakfast, why don't you try having just two glasses of wine with your evening meal?' Why, thank you! We are all cured.

Besides, I had ADHD, even though I didn't know it, so 'plans' and 'routines' were kryptonite to me.

OCD was never mentioned in my bulimia 'therapy'. I hadn't thought to tell the therapist that when I was 12 I washed my hands with bleach until they bled and if anyone put outdoor clothes on my bed, I had to change my bedding. I had begun to mutter little mantras, strict routines like 'blink five times before you wash your hands, then blink ten times after you have dried them'. If my blinks were interrupted in any way, I would start it all from the beginning.

I wonder, if I had kept on seeing the therapist, if she would have unearthed this stuff, found a connection between that and my disordered eating and chaotic thinking. In my twenties, the internet was still new and clunky to use. I was desperate for help, but there was none of the instant access we have now, where with a couple of clicks you can get information about obsessive-compulsive disorder, bulimia, ADHD or what a Chihuahua crossed with a Great Dane looks like.

The therapist and I never got there. I sat in the hall of the little clinic in Acton looking forward to my fourth session, but she stood me up. Eventually her colleague came along to tell me she was very sorry, but that she must have forgotten.

'Oh, that's okay! I have loads to do anyway!' I said breezily, trying to save face.

Now I am almost 50, my heart breaks at how easily young people accept being let down. The word 'entitled' is thrown around a lot to denigrate a young person who is confident and able to ask for what they need. Which is exactly what I wish I could have done. Now, I would ask to be referred to someone else. But when I was young, I did not feel entitled to being looked after. It was all my own fault for *needing* therapy. I was putting the therapist out by being a client. I was all take, take, take. I imagined everyone at the little clinic in Acton thinking, *Look at her, draining NHS resources because she can't stop eating cake. She's meant to be bulimic but she's fat! She can't even do an eating disorder right!*

In no way did I blame her for not turning up. I imagined my therapist was in a pub instead, telling all her cool friends what a loser I was. Therapists train for years, work really hard, and the least you could do as a client was to not bother them with your problems. Why did I imagine I was worthy of being helped? I left. I didn't go back, and I didn't ask my GP to refer me to someone else.

This experience should not put anyone off getting therapy, just to be clear. If a dodgy plumber fails to unblock your loo, you don't just let it overflow until you are swimming in poo. You find another plumber – maybe this time one you have researched or got a recommendation for. Not that I am saying my therapist was dodgy. I mean you need to try different therapists, perhaps different therapy practices, to see which one works for you.

Though I know that when you are in a fog of addiction, or OCD or ADHD or whatever, which has led you to seek help from a therapist in the first place, this is easier said than done. When you are in a funk, it is easy to get derailed altogether from moving towards recovery and asking for help. This may look like a lack of willpower, but I believe it is misdirected willpower.

I thought lack of willpower was what was keeping me locked into bulimia. It turns out I have an abundance of it. The time commitment and effort addicts make takes real dedication. How else would we repeatedly do something which harms us and those who love us? How else do we tolerate being seen as unreliable, holding ourselves back, acting against our own values? We are *driven*.

For years, decades, I believed I needed to stop puking; that was the only problem. I didn't realise that throwing up was just the tip of the iceberg. It was the obsessive thoughts about food and physically not being able to stop eating once I started – *those* were the problem. It was my desperate need to pause the motor in my brain but not understanding the first thing about why it was there or what it did. The problem started long before I put my head in a toilet bowl.

I told Christian what I was doing. By this time, I was 31. I had been doing stand-up for eight years but had not got beyond 'promising new act' and I certainly wasn't earning a living from it. I was still life modelling. Christian and I went for a walk in Princes Street Gardens the day after a gig in Edinburgh. We'd been booked at the club for the whole weekend. We sat and talked, sitting on the hill in the sunshine. He told me that he'd been a heavy smoker for years and couldn't give up. He said he'd wanted to be a comedian but it felt so hard to imagine a career like that was possible, but when he gave up smoking, he knew he'd be able to do it.

'Giving up smoking was the Impossible Thing,' he said to me. 'I realised that if I couldn't imagine a life with cigarettes, I couldn't imagine myself being a comic. When I did finally give up, it made comedy seem possible because I had already done *the* Impossible Thing.'

I understood suddenly, for the first time, that bulimia was *my* Impossible Thing. Sure, smoking was more socially acceptable. No one says in a restaurant 'I'm just off for a puke', but in essence, in the context of 'the thing I need to do before I can live my life' it was the same thing. Realising this was possible was huge.

That weekend, I found the words to tell Christian about the extent of my bulimia. It came tumbling out – how debilitating it was, how wretched it made me feel. He was not shocked. In fact, he told me of someone else he had known who had been bulimic. This blew my mind. Other people who did this existed? Of course I knew they did, otherwise it wouldn't have a name, but they were usually people I read about in magazines or ones agony aunts talked about on TV. The relief of telling someone made me feel hope, actual hope, that one day my life would not be shackled by this horrible cycle of bingeing and purging.

Starting to talk to people about it was how I finally found the 12-step groups for compulsive overeaters. I went to my first one in a church hall in central London. I've always liked church halls. They take me back to happy days of Brownies and ballet classes, comforting little kitchens with tins of custard creams.

At this meeting, people sat around and a chairperson asked, 'Are there any newcomers?' I put my hand up.

'Welcome,' said everyone.

I looked around at the other people in this circle. They were young and old, men and women, smartly dressed, mostly. It was a lunchtime meeting so they had come from work.

There is a rule in 12-step groups that whoever you see, whatever you hear, it stays in the room when you leave. So I can't tell you much about what was said in the meeting and what people shared, all beginning with, 'My name is blah-de-blah and I'm a compulsive overeater.' But I will tell you how my heart wept with relief being among people who understood, who were or had been a compulsive overeater. These people weren't weirdos; they were intelligent, kind people who, like me, understood that buffets were the work of the devil and that their lives were blighted by the existence of them.

They talked about triggers and feelings and 'checking in' with themselves. Every time one of them opened their mouth to share I found new acceptance and understanding. Tiny, simple things people said were so relatable that they made me giggle.

'I had to give something I bought back to John Lewis. It was stressing me out,' this man shared. 'I kept putting it off. The stress was making me want to binge. I called my sponsor. It really helped. I realised it wasn't going to be John Lewis *himself* dealing with my refund.'

This. This! Little worries like this mounted up in my head and made me binge rather than get on with dealing with them. My friends and family couldn't understand. 'You locked yourself in the house and made yourself sick all day because you couldn't face returning some socks?' But here, people GOT that. The word 'triggered' has been so mocked and misused in the world of social media that it's almost lost its original, serious meaning. Sometimes people say you are 'triggered' in order to demean you, without understanding the very real psychological phenomenon. Because actually, being triggered is a response to trauma, a debilitating experience for those of us who are neurodivergent, have anxiety, suffer from PTSD, are addicts or those who have been traumatised by others through words or actions.

When I was in 12-step group meetings, we often talked about triggers. They are the things that give you the push towards self-harm, whatever that might be – drugs, booze, food, whatever it is you do to quieten your anxiety. Learning what they are is tremendously useful. I have learned that two of my triggers are admin/having to open post and feta cheese.

Other people in the group mentioned ADHD and slowly it began to dawn on me that OCD, ADHD and other brain stuff may be contributing to my bulimia. But I was not ready to investigate further. I have been avoiding using the word 'journey' as I don't want to sound like a self-help app, but the very notion that it may be my brain, rather than purely my emotions, that was leading me to act out compulsions took me many years to understand. But still, my life was changed by going to 12-step meetings, even though the ADHD piece of the puzzle was missing. For now, I was just basking in the utter joy of finally finding myself, for whole days, then whole weeks, not bingeing or throwing up. It was freedom: it was, finally, a life!

DOPAMINE NIGHTS

Comedy comes in all forms: theatre, sitcoms, films. I loved them all, but the only one I had a desperate need to *do* was stand-up comedy. Given what we have discussed so far, it doesn't take a genius to work out why. Yes, that's right: it requires very little admin and zero technical requirements other than to stand in the light, talk into the mike, and try to face the audience.

With my ADHD impulsivity, recklessness and inability to think of consequences or follow instructions, stand-up comedy was the only thing I wanted to do. The only way I could hope to make a decent living. It was where all the rules were my own, and however wretched the feeling when it went wrong, only I was affected by it. There was no boss, no colleagues, no one to get cross with me. Obviously there was the soul-sucking horror of dying on stage, but even that was preferable to writing a CV.

Would I still have put myself into the lion's den of the open-spot comedy circuit if my ADHD had been diagnosed and treated when I was a child? Would I if I had been able to switch off that ADHD motor, which endlessly drove me towards electrifying risk? What would have been the attraction, to this bonkers career choice which meant no social life outside of the industry for years, and had no guarantee of ever earning me a living? It's an endless chase for a high, so that you feel connected, alive.

Perhaps it's simply a more comforting thought to imagine I would not have become a stand-up at all had I been aware of my ADHD. Truth is, I reckon that if I had been diagnosed early, I would still have become a comic, but a better one, a more focused one. Maybe I'd have had more fun. I might have been one of those comics who recorded their sets, listened back, made changes for the better and didn't stick around to get smashed with people they had just met. Stand-up gave me an identity, long before I became a comedian. I watched Billy Connolly and Richard Pryor, Joan Rivers and Victoria Wood, and thought *These are my people.* Maybe everyone feels like an outsider as a child, but only a certain kind of personality is bothered by it to such an extent that they build a career which ensures they are the center of attention. I relied on my big brother a lot, clung on to him when I was small, so when we went to different high schools, I found it tough.

I flitted around socially, but never found a tribe. I even tried to be a goth at one point in my teens. It's very hard to get your skin pale enough when you're an Asian goth. I tried to do it using flour and water. When it dried, my face cracked and I had too much of a 'bakery' vibe, which the goths did not embrace. Socially I was 'too much', too in your face, needy, a 'try hard'. I couldn't slot myself into a conversation naturally because I couldn't help interrupting, changing the subject, blurting out something weird or trying to crack jokes without having made a connection. In short, I was socially dying on my arse before I had even got onto a stage. Good unintentional practise for a comic.

Often, it's not being one of the popular kids that makes you want to be a stand-up. Feeling ignored, undermined and underestimated can lead to the desire to have a voice, to be 'famous' in some way. Anyone can feel like that, whether or not that person has ADHD.

When I was a child and experienced racism, fame felt like it would protect me from it. Anybody who has ever been bullied might have also experienced this feeling of wanting to 'be' somebody, so people can't hurt you. 'I want to be famous' might sound like, 'I think I am so fantastic that everyone should know about ME!' But for most, it comes from a tender part of yourself that wants acceptance but has not been attended to, has been neglected. 'I feel invisible and voiceless, and I want to be famous so I am visible and have a voice' is more accurate.

My father, a renowned satirist and poet who enjoyed huge fame in our native Iran, had his own version of this. It surprised me when my grandmother said, 'He was a very quiet child.' This is often the case with famous people. They are rarely the 'stand-out' one as children, the confident ones.

On a rare occasion I was able get my father to talk about his childhood, he told me his name isn't actually Hadi. His name had originally been Nasser. Hadi had been the name of his older brother, who had died when he was two. This was rural Iran, infant deaths were common, and my grandparents hadn't registered my father's birth. They used his dead older brother's birth certificate to enrol him in school.

'So', my father said, 'at school they called me Hadi. I did not understand why that was my name. At home they called me Nasser. My father died; I was six and was sent away to a charity boarding school. Nasser did not exist anymore. I did not exist anymore. I thought, *I am going to be famous so everybody knows I exist.* And by his early twenties, he was.

So there are gentle reasons, sad reasons, for people wanting to be famous. The brilliant comedian Arnold Brown has one of my favourite lines about why we go into stand-up: 'I became a comedian because of the lack of attention I got as an adult.'

How did people get noticed? Fit in? How did I have to act, to make people want to include me? As I got older, these feelings turned into hypersensitivity. If people laughed across the park then they were definitely laughing at me. *They think I'm an idiot/ugly/uncool* – or, more specifically, *They have* found out *I'm an idiot/ugly/uncool.* The people laughing probably didn't even know I was there.

When, as a teen and a young adult (and still, occasionally, as an older adult. I don't know why I am pretending to you that I am 'cured' of being hypersensitive. It still creeps up on me from time to time), a friend didn't call me back, well, that was that: 'They hate me. They answered the calls of every other friend except for me. They are thinking, *God, she is annoying, why does she think I like her?*' Did these thoughts stop me calling them again? No. I would leave several messages. Then carry on obsessing over why they had still not called back: *They might not have got the messages. They are grossed out by me because I've left too many messages. They hate me. Stop calling. Don't call!* Locked into these obsessive negative thoughts, I would call. Again and again.

I wasn't always paranoid; often I *was* being ghosted. I attached myself to people who were not good friends, but they were exciting, fun. They woke my ADHD brain up. They brought chaos and dopamine, and eventually hurtful lows, because this chemical reaction was not friendship. It was a high. It took me a long time to figure that out.

I talked about this once to my son. He was about nine and having a tricky time with a friend who was excluding him. 'Friendship is a job!' I declared. 'Just because someone is fun and funny and exciting to hang out with, it doesn't mean they are good at the job of being a friend.' I carried on, enjoying imparting my knowledge to my child. 'A friend is someone who cares how you are feeling, considers your feelings. If they don't, it doesn't mean they are deliberately trying to make you feel bad. It just means they haven't learned to be a good friend.'

'How old were you,' my son asked, 'when you realised this? When you stopped having friends who made you feel bad?'

That knocked me off my 'wise mummy' perch. 'Erm, about thirty-three, darling. Let's get some ice cream!'

This cycle I got into of being drawn to people who would be inconsistent with me, who made friends with me then ghosted me, carried on as I got older, and it became boyfriend or potential new boyfriend whose call I was waiting for. I held my breath, paused my life until they called, which would give me that dopamine hit.

These relationships were not thought through. Pros and cons were not weighed up; no thought did I give to what my needs were and whether they were being met. Everything was a 'DON'T LOOK! JUST JUMP!' gamble, a risk.

When I lost, and it hurt, I'd take the gamble again and again because if they *did* call, if they *did* turn up, the relief, the high, was immense.

What I went through to become a successful stand-up comedian – the fear, the rejection, being booed off stage, being heckled to tears, the feeling of *Oh God, everyone hates me* – was another version of this wretched gamble. I took it knowing the relief when it went well was worth it. Up, up, up, then down, down, down, down – an endless, high-octane fairground ride. It was like being drawn to touch an electric fence when you *know* it is an electric fence (something which I have done and strongly advise against. It *did* keep me out of a field but I'm almost certain I saw a sheep mouth the word *moron*).

In stand-up, this relief after putting yourself up to be rejected comes in the form of laughter from the audience. Even if I died on my arse ten times in a row, eventually I would connect and they would laugh. And it was like blood-letting; that was the high. I trusted it would happen eventually; no matter how bad I felt and for how long, that trust never went.

I made friends with Arthur Smith when I was still a fledgling comedian. We went for a drink together one day in the bar at the Royal Court Theatre. As we walked down the

King's Road, a couple of young guys smiled at him and said, 'You're Arthur Smith, you're brilliant!'

Arthur smiled as we walked on, looked back at them and said, 'Thank you, sirs, as are you.'

'What's it like?' I asked him. 'Being famous?'

He said, 'Well, my level of fame is perfect. I'm just famous enough for the world to be a little bit friendlier. I walk down the street and occasionally I get a cheerful "hello" from a stranger. It's lovely.'

That's what I wanted. I wanted the world to be just a little bit friendlier. A place where people let me play, and where occasionally, a stranger might say 'hello'.

Risk and ADHD go hand in hand. If you are unable to stay focused, or even just awake, unless you are excited, the impulsivity can lead to great decisions and terrible ones. Some are antisocial. For example, running across railway tracks, criminal behaviour and interrupting a conversation to launch into a story about yourself (by far the worst). *My risk-taking when I was younger took the form of doing jokes and impersonations at my parents' frequent parties. Making everyone laugh by standing there and saying stuff petrified and intoxicated me. The gamble was a thrill, like I was jump-starting myself.*

'Funny' was what boys were expected to be; girls were meant to be the audience for the guys. I saw it, throughout my teens, among the in-crowd: the girls looked cool and elegant and the boys showed off, being funny. It was annoying.

Taking risks feeds ADHD's need for stimulation. It gave me the top-up my dopamine-deficient brain craved. A few times in my teens, shyness overtook me to the extent that I had to leave the party I was at. But as my confidence grew (otherwise known as 'discovering alcohol'), if I was at a party or hanging out and someone was being funny, I loved it. I was entertained. When no one was holding court, unable to stand stillness, I would step up and do it. My insides would fizz and I couldn't be quiet. I would be noisy, do impressions, be exuberant, gabble away to strangers.

This, to me, was a bigger risk than it would be to many, thanks to my hypersensitivity. Sometimes, people would think me a delight and we'd connect and I would be a social hit. Other times, they found me annoying, too much, hogging a space and not letting anyone else get a word in. I carried on like an out-of-control springer spaniel, convinced I'd find a way to win over these people who clearly couldn't stand me.

A gambling addict doesn't stop when they've lost. They keep going. The stakes need to be big if you are a risk-taker. To get the high you crave, the consequences really have to burn. Comedians, gamblers and opportunist burglars have a lot in common. My ADHD-related spontaneity means I can roll with change and am insatiably up for new experiences with new people. Lack of spontaneity makes me gloomy, so I am suited to stand-up comedy, where spontaneity can happen at any moment and I have no problem bending with it. I need it. It keeps me alert, keeps me interested, hyperfocused.

Risk is, well, risky, but it can also mean you follow your dreams. Not in a 'So strong, babes! SLAY, QUEEN!' way, but because you are simply incapable of doing anything else.

You feel like the misfit, the odd one out. You are hurt by things that seem like water off a duck's back for other people who don't lie in bed for days with anxiety because an acquaintance passed them in the street and didn't say 'hello' as enthusiastically as they did. On the comedy circuit, you are among other misfits, so it feels more comfortable. You are with other people who flit wildly from subject to subject, interrupting conversations, blurting out inappropriate things, desperate to tell you their thoughts and their story. You are with fellows who are, like you, very sensitive *and* bloody flaky, who get wrapped up in their own world and forget what it was they promised you they would do for you. They understand that unspoken need you have to be a comic and they know what you put yourself through to be a good one. You are with people who can be wildly exuberant then completely distant in the same five minutes, people for whom 'over-sharing' is just a normal chat, who take chaos in their stride, and there is never an inappropriate time to crack a joke. In short, it is backstage at *The Muppet Show*.

ADHD is rife amongst the self-employed, particularly in creative industries, particularly comedians. Now that I know the signs I'm like the kid from *The Sixth Sense*: 'I see ADHD people!' Soon, I think, we will have a comedian writing a book about what it was like being diagnosed as *not* having ADHD.

People are very quick to say to comics, 'You are so brave, I could never do it, I'd be so scared.' You wouldn't say to a boxer, 'Oh God, I *couldn't* do what you do! I'd be so scared of getting punched!' You don't want to be a boxer. And that's okay.

Dying on stage is called dying for a reason. It hollows you out. Your very soul has escaped the humiliation by jumping out of your body and off a cliff. You die in front of potential agents, TV and radio producers, your parents. In front of large audiences and small. Dying a death on stage is different from having a bad gig. You can resurrect a clunky gig and you can have a laugh with the other comics about a bad one, but a death is a long, lonely howl into the mouth of hell. There are extraordinarily funny people in all walks of life, but a stand-up comedian is a different animal. A stand-up comedian is someone who dies on their arse, feels that horror, and yet does not consider giving it up to become a florist. To put yourself through this again and again means that stand-up comedy isn't something you *want* to do; it's something you *need* to do. When I was still a very new comic, I got booed off stage. This is different to dying or being booed by one or two people. This is when the whole audience, en masse, boo until you walk off. It happened in Belfast, at The Belfast Empire. I had never been to Belfast before; I had only ever read about it. I was travelling *on a plane* to a gig. *This is what it must be like to be Bono*, I thought. Patrick Kielty was compèring and he was as home at the Empire as I was unfamiliar with it. Backstage, another comic on the bill was also in the tiny corridor we stood in before the show, performing vigorous, strangely audible press-ups, then getting up and rapping full throttle along to the music in his Walkman. No pre-show group hugs in stand-up. It left no room for me to gather my thoughts or prepare myself mentally, let alone do any pre-show press-ups.

'God, I'm so nervous,' I said to a guy who worked there, mostly so I could just splutter some words out of my mouth before I went on stage. The man was not the nurturing type. He shrugged, and said, 'They'll hate you. You're English, you're a woman and you're ethnic.' Kielty was about to introduce me; I had no time to change any of these things. I walked on stage with all the swagger a terrified, English, ethnic woman could muster.

I did okay for 40 seconds. I got laughs. Some women in the audience looked encouragingly at me, the way you might at a duckling about to go for a swim in a lake of crocodiles. But then it flipped. One *boo*, two *boo*s, then a whoosh of *boo*s from all over the big room, all connecting to make one huge, relentless 'BOOOOOO!' They hated me.

In the moment, it doesn't feel real. I was quite calm, smiling, laughing even, shouting back a bit. It was almost exhilarating while I was still on stage; it was a kind of shock, like it was happening to someone else. But it was definitely me. They definitely hated me. It was once I walked off the stage, was back on the floor, in the club, that my body reacted to what happened and began to shake a little. I was, however, absolutely determined not to let it show on my face that I was bothered. Huge smile, ignore the shaking. Go to the bar.

The worst had happened. This was the big risk. I was exactly where I feared ending up every time I stepped onto a stage. I was in the horror, and I was not going to run away. Nope. I was a stand-up comedian and I was going to have a drink. I was not going to let any fucker think I was going to run away, though that was exactly what I wanted to do. I forced my body to obey me and stay.

It was the interval and I was in a throng of people who had just booed me off. I was in the middle of a hate pie. Some ignored me and just laughed at me with friends. Lovely. I was bringing people together. Some told me I was shit again, just in case I had thought I'd stormed it. A few told me, 'Fair play to you, you've got some balls sticking around.' And I did. I did indeed have balls and they had taken quite the kicking. I needed to stick around for a drink, to smile and laugh along. I took a risk that night; I was warned the odds were against me; I did it anyway. And I would do it again in another club, in front of another audience, the very next night, and the night after. This is the difference between someone who is just funny, and a stand-up comedian. Anyone can make their friends laugh, but to bomb like I just had, in front of strangers, and absolutely not rethink your career choices? That's when you're a comic. One who more than likely has ADHD.

I should have gone back to my hotel straight away; breathed. I didn't need to prove anything to that audience. Leaving the building is what a person with balanced brain chemicals would do. But my brain pathways were desperate for a drink to slow them down. My first thought once

I was pouring booze down me was, *This will not make me give up.* I didn't want to let anyone see how devastated I was. It was not the best for me, staying out drinking that night. But my chaotic head was powerless not to obey my motor. It was impossible for me to take a breath and think any further than that impulse. I wish ADHD spontaneity had made me spontaneously go back to my hotel sober, call a friend and meditate. But back then, mindfulness, processing and self-care were not even in my vocabulary. Even if they had been, they take a degree of responsibility to implement, and that was unthinkable.

So that's the risk, that hundreds of strangers will simultaneously decide that you are shit at your job and pretty much worthless, and make sure you know this. The risk was also that established comedians and promoters would spread the news of my death on the circuit, which they did, with embellishments. (In one account I heard years later, a comic said, 'Oh yeah! You got booed off in Belfast because you called the audience terrorists!' No. I did not say any such thing. I was actually doing an Anne Robinson impression. But I think I prefer people to believe I made that Belfast audience boo me off by screaming 'YOU'RE ALL A BUNCH OF TERROR-ISTS.' It's more rock and roll than the reality: I was doing a hack impersonation of a teatime game show host.)

For those of us who felt left out or ignored when we were children, stand-up comedy is the second time at the playground. It's something I had the recklessness to do, that all the people who underestimated me or bullied me cannot do. When you make people laugh, for that moment, you are great friends. You are smashing a gig not when you are getting smatterings of guffaws here and there – they are not satisfying gigs – but when you not only connect with the audience, but the audience members connect with one another, so the crowd becomes one huge, loud, beautiful monster roaring with laughter back at you in giant waves, crashing joy over your stage. That's the real delight. That feeling takes away all the frustration, all the doubt, all the anxiety you have carried and you are, for a while, euphoric: anything is possible and you are completely at one with yourself. A quicker way to do this of course is with crack, but the pay is not as good.

You need to get experience to get to this place, of course, and loads of time. You have to put in hours and hours, years, into becoming reliably bulletproof. You have to be obsessed with it to stick it out.

My first-ever gig was in a room above the Camden Head pub in Islington. I counted the people in the audience. Twelve, including my brother and my cousin. But to me, it might as well have been the Super Bowl. I had never felt this level of nerves before. I didn't know it was *possible* to feel this level of nerves and still be standing. I thought, *The compère is going to introduce me in a minute and my legs feel like jelly. There is no way they will be able to carry me to the stage. I will just collapse.* The nerves are shocking. Seriously. I worry they will shorten my life. I was on with another comic called Brian Higgins who was Scottish and warm and friendly, which I appreciated. There was another brand-new comic on the bill that night who was from Bristol: Steven Merchant. He sensibly decided stand-up was a bonkers thing to do and went off and wrote *The Office* and *Extras* with Ricky Gervais instead.

The gig went okay. The audience laughed and I was not booed off. It was the most incredible night of my life. The promoter gave me a fiver. A fiver! I was paid! Brian gave me a wooden cherry for 'popping your comedy cherry'. I have no idea why he had a wooden cherry on him but it added to the magic of that first night.

I was hit-and-miss as a comedian for years. More than most. I did pretty much no preparation and left it all to chance each night. I could do nothing in the day if I had a gig in the evening but pace and fret. I told myself that how well I did depended on my 'mojo'. That was just what I was like; I was rock and roll! I had no idea that rock and roll stars actually have a serious work ethic and respect their talent. Rock stars are serious geeks. Bruce Springsteen does not turn up to his gigs and say, 'Oh, I dunno! I'll just see how it does! If it all goes to shit, I'll just get pissed after!' I was just bouncing around the comedy circuit, from gig to gig – some good, some awful – with no plan, no idea of how to push myself forward. Writing new material was impossible, because I had a five-minute set that worked and I could not let go of it. It was like I was clinging on to the edge of a cliff and that five minutes was all I had to hold on to. I treated stand-up like a drug, not a profession. My manic mind, my ADHD anxiety had a few moments of respite on stage when I felt present.

I chatted to the audience a lot. That was what I enjoyed. I didn't have to have a structure, or a plan.

Everyone has their own idea of what being 'famous' and 'successful' means. I always know who is going to be huge, who is more businesslike and who, like me, is still shuffling around in the playground happy to be included. I was on a televised show with Sarah Millican at the Edinburgh Festival once. She sat in the wings, scribbling diligently in her notebook, getting her head together before the recording. I sauntered along with a beer, chatting away to people, not thinking about my set. Telling myself 'I am old school; I trust my mojo.' Leaving everything to chance? Well, I was a comic, not an accountant, right? 'That's just how I work, I take risks, I am up for the gamble!' I told myself. But really, I was unable to be like Sarah, unable to sit quietly and gather my thoughts.

Jimmy Carr also started at the same time as me. At a time when comedy was still quite a 'punk' thing to do, the circuit attracted people like me who wanted to be away from the mainstream, liked to be on the move and were really into getting pissed after the show. Jimmy wasn't like that. Jimmy was businesslike; Jimmy had a Filofax. In the 1990s and early 2000s, a Filofax was the armour of the organised, the professional, the person who takes their career seriously. He quickly became known as being the one who did the most open spots, trying to get reliable enough to get paid. He drove around London, turning up at clubs on the chance they might let him on. He had had a proper, well-paid job before he went into comedy. He expected comedy to give him a good income, eventually. We were chatting backstage at a gig once and he mentioned that ours was a 'recession-proof business'. 'Haha-hahaha!' I said to my friends later. 'Who thinks of this as a business? Hahahahaha!' Future millionaires, clearly.

I could not think that way. I could not think much beyond the day I was in. Jimmy, and others like him, who were better able to harness their talent early on, navigated the industry. They seemed to effortlessly schmooze while I sank pints at the bar, chatting to people and disappearing off into a boozy night with them, giving off the air that I was not serious about my career. Dopamine over career, every time.

Another comic who was kicking around at the time and was a massive gossip said to me one day, 'Jimmy told me he thinks you're good but you haven't got any focus.' Jimmy was damn right. I knew it but I couldn't do anything about it because my brain was clinging onto the roof of a train hurtling along at full speed, usually in the wrong direction. You can see where you *should* be going, but you can't get off; it's too fast and although the speed is terrifying, jumping is not an option. I didn't want to be performing hit-and-miss gigs in rooms above pubs for the rest of my career, but this horrific anxiety lurking inside me was triggered by the slight-est thing, interfering with any chance I had to focus.

The truth was, in fact, that I cannot focus until I am physically on the stage. I wish I could be like the businesslike comics. They were the geeks I aspired to be at school; those who did their homework the day it was set. I was the kid that fretted and panicked, rushing through as best I could on the bus on the way to school. I still could not sit down and do my homework. The only time I could plan my material, the only time I could think of jokes, was when I was actually onstage. And all the reviews came back with 'does not fulfil her potential'.

Since my diagnosis and therapy, I understand the extra support my brain needs. I work differently now, with none of the overwhelming anxiety. I make time in my day to write material for my shows. I record every gig when I'm making a new set. I won't ever listen to it again, I accept this, so I pay someone else to transcribe it. I can skim through the waffle and find the places where I had done new stuff, remember what worked and keep it in for next time. For twenty years I winged it. Finally, I am starting to do my homework and it shows in my performance. Better late than never. (Poor old ADHD cannot be blamed for everything, though. It is possible to have it *and* not leave your career to chance.)

Bizarrely, everyone seemed focused on their own career rather than mine. I never found that one friend on the comedy circuit who told me what I was meant to be doing, where I was meant to be, like I had at school. There were very few women on the circuit for me to cling to. There was a cluster of women who were a little older than me who just gave me 'mean girl' vibes. Though they could just have been constipated. I didn't have the internet back then to search *how not to feel massively insecure and self-conscious in the company of other human beings.*

The fact that I wasn't white became a 'thing' again. People kept bringing it up. Every single journalist asked me, 'So you're Iranian?! WHAT do your parents think about what you do?'

'They are very disappointed because they *really* wanted me to be a trapeze artist,' I would say, but they never let it go. Agents and producers, the gatekeepers to the industry, made it clear that my not being white was my Unique Selling Point, though I never woke up in the morning and thought, *Oh look! I'm brown! Again!* I didn't, couldn't, look deeper into it. The conversation around this kind of thing didn't exist like it does now. It's hard to explain to newer comics how different the landscape of comedy was back then. I was in my twenties and the fact that I was a woman stand-up and not white would either make people go, 'OH MY GOD YOU ARE SO BRAVE! THIS IS AMAZING' or they would say 'ALL SHE TALKS ABOUT IS BEING A WOMAN AND BROWN' or occasionally 'Can I get you a drink? I'm really into P*ki girls' (to be fair, the last one happened just the once, but bizarrely once is enough for it to stay with you).

It was a lot to deal with, and so I didn't deal with it. The second I stepped off the stage, I went to the bar. I drank so much after gigs that the next day was a blur of anxiety and regret. My career 'plan' was to have no plan whatsoever and say 'yes!' to everything without considering how utterly unsuited I was to it.

'Can you host *Sing-a-Long-a-Sound of Music* at Croydon Clocktower?'

'YES!'

I had never sung in public before. I had never watched *The Sound of Music* to the end. I always fell asleep once the nun and the grumpy bloke got it together. I did not research it; I did not dress up. I did not know the audience dressed up. In short, I did not know what *Sing-a-Long-a-Sound of Music* was. With only an open-spot stage experience, I got up in front of hundreds of people dressed as Nazis and brown paper packages tied up with string.

I had to do some stand-up to warm them up. I did not have the experience to 'work the room'; I just had my club set. I'm not sure how much the Nazis and the brown paper packages tied up with string enjoyed my material about my Iranian grandmother's obsession with pomegranates. They looked baffled and remained very, very quiet. The producer of the show, panicking that I was bombing, mouthed and mimed, 'Sing! Sing!' I began to sing 'My Favourite Things'. After a fairly robust start, I found I only knew the first four lines, so I sang them, twice and glanced over to the producer who seemed to be having some kind of seizure. *I'd better start the film*, I thought, considering a third rendition a bit much. I announced, to a hall full of hardcore Maria fans, 'Now let's all go to the Alps of Switzerland!' If you have never had a crowd of people dressed as nuns crossly screeching, 'It's AUSTRIA!!' at you, you haven't lived. I did not stop to get paid. I just went home.

My audiences were, at that point in my career, more confident than me. This was a problem seeing as I needed this career to work because I knew I would not, could not, ever get it together to write a CV to apply for jobs.

I had to get an agent. Unfortunately, I had the same reaction to agents as I had done to maths teachers: 'I'm an idiot; you know everything. You're going to tell me off, aren't you?' I was taken on by an agent who sent me off to a cognitive behavioural therapist to work on my confidence. He guessed I wasn't all that confident when he shouted at me in front of all his staff and I burst into tears. With modern eyes, I suppose some would say, 'if you shout at people in front of your staff you've got the problem' but back then, I was the one who was sent to a therapist. It did work. I stopped crying when my agent bellowed at me. I also learned to manage my nerves in big rowdy rooms. I became a 'big rowdy room' comic, a proper club comic, and I remain very proud of that. I loved it. Going out in front of a crowd that might turn on you if you don't grab them straight away and nailing it was exhilarating. I loved it. It was like bloodletting. I became a proper, gladiatorial, machine-gun-fire comic. I believe it was The Fresh Prince who said, 'My life is a cage and on stage I'm free.' There was never anywhere I wanted to be more than in a rowdy comedy club, watching other acts and risking dying on my arse.

Stand-up comedy is a fast-evolving medium. The gladiatorial-style comedy performed in bear pits is not so popular with new generations, who prefer the gentle performers that have begun to talk more about their feelings and the issues of the day. 'Honest' and 'thought-provoking'. Critics have begun to judge a show not by the laughs, but by the comedian's 'message'. This type of comedy attracts a different audience, who were much more likely to bring a book with them to read during the interval than a large inflatable penis.

There is room for everybody, I say, but I am a comedy nerd and get excited when there is a buzz about a new comic and a rush to watch them. Apart from loving the comedy, I want to see where they are taking the medium. It inspires me. I have never felt like an 'old hand'; stand-up always feels fresh if you move with it. That said, I am dismayed when 'club comic' is used as a derisory term and often comes prefixed with 'just a'. Richard Pryor was thought-provoking, but he came up through the spit-and-sawdust clubs. He was a club comic.

Let me tell you about club comics. Club comics rip the living shit out of a room, whether the people in it are university educated or not. A club comic does not need the audience to have anything in common with them. You can plonk a club comic in any venue, anywhere in the country and they will work their butt off to make that audience laugh for as long and as hard as possible, whether or not they share their values or listen to the same podcasts. A club comic is the foot soldier of the entertainment industry, so if you hear a performer haughtily say, 'I don't want to just go into a room and make groups of drunk stags and hens laugh' what they mean is, 'I *can't* do that. It is terrifying, I will wet myself. For God's sake, some of them are working class!' (If you think that I have plonked this rant in my book just to vent about snobbery in the comedy industry, which has nothing to do with ADHD, you would be right.)

Early in my career, my agent had a policy of never calling club promoters to get me gigs. Some would call this bad
business, and indeed it got me in into £8,000 of debt, but I
went along with it because by this time, he had made me feel
my success lay in his hands. So the only clubs I played were
in the Jongleurs chain. These were huge, well-paid rooms up
and down the country which encouraged birthday parties
and stag and hen nights. These groups can be tough, because
often it's just one or two of the people in the party who want
to see comedy. The rest just came because they had to, and
just got bladdered. They looked the same as I did when I was
forced to watch a male stripper hired for a friend's twenty-first
birthday party. I was awkward. I stared at my feet thinking,
*HE IS NAKED! WHY AM I THE ONLY ONE WHO FINDS
THIS STRANGE IN YOUR NAN'S HOUSE?* For some, it will
be the first and last time they will ever go to see live comedy.
The Jongleurs clubs were nightclubs. The crowd would get
very drunk then the tables were folded away for the disco
afterwards. I loved them.

I am proud I learned how to conquer rooms like those.
They were honest: no frills, no airs, nothing fancy, just
comedy and fried chicken in a basket with a disco afterwards.
No one came to see a specific comic. You got no respect
from the audience until you'd earned it. In fact, it was mostly
naked hostility until you shut them down and proved yourself, especially if you were a woman and especially if you were
an un-white woman. My ADHD was my asset at these clubs:
the instinct to shrink away was overridden by my need to

jump into an adrenaline pit of fire. Every atom inside me was FULLY ENGAGED, utterly alert. It was freedom. The adrenaline coursed through me for hours afterwards. Then I would need it again and again. There was no party, no date, no wedding that was more important than a gig. 'What a shame you can't come to my thirtieth!' No, it's not a shame I can't come to your very special event, because I am going to be in a smoky basement somewhere, making drunk strangers laugh. There is no better way to spend an evening.

Jongleurs would book you for a whole weekend and pay for your hotel. There would be two shows on Friday and Saturday night. The older acts called them 'mortgage payers'. Not that I was anywhere near getting a mortgage. They were the only clubs I played and not every weekend. I wasn't on the normal circuit. It wasn't working out with the agent. It slowly began to dawn on me that it wasn't normal to have an agent who regularly tore strips off you and told you your show was 'the worst I have ever seen'. It makes me sad when I remember how long it took me to object to being treated like this. It's only now I can look back and see how eroded my self-esteem had become, how I was drawn to agents, friends and men who in one breath praised me to the skies and in the next made sure I knew I was a sodding disappointment who needed to change everything about themselves in order to be worthy of their attention. Anxiety smothers everything. And when you have ADHD you find it hard to be still and effectively process things, so you push it all down, hide it away, carry on until something quite unrelated makes you have a screaming fit at your boyfriend and, just off the top of my head, lob a full, family-sized carton of toffee-flavoured yoghurt at the wall.

I hung on miserably at the agency until it came to a head for a few of the other comics there too and they left. I crept out after them. I went with a different agent, one who considered getting me work as part of his job.

Why did it take me so long to go? Because my brain only has 'compliant' or 'JUMP' modes. I cannot channel my energy to stand up for myself until I am against a wall, until it is make or break time.

I was 31 at this point. I had been in 12-step recovery for a few months and for the first time since I was a teenager, I wasn't in the fog of food: I was eating three meals a day and not bingeing or throwing up. I had a life. I could have meals out with friends and actually enjoy myself. I didn't disappear to the toilet immediately after meals *and* (this is huge) I could share a Twix. No problem. It was euphoric.

My new agent filled my diary. Not leaving things to chance this time, I put together a tight set and made it bullet-proof. No experimenting, no faffing around with the crowd, just putting out my best 10 or 20 minutes. It worked. Reports came back to my agent that I was smashing it and could I come back? 'YES!'

I had done a show at the Edinburgh Festival in 2003. My old, shouty agent had thought it best to not put my name, venue or time of the show on my Edinburgh poster – 'It'll create intrigue,' he insisted. So there were just pictures of my face plastered all over Edinburgh with no information. People had to guess who I was, what I did, where I was performing and at what time. Remarkably, this, and the fact that I hadn't written a show before, made for a pretty disastrous run. Now though, it was 2006. I was in love, I was puke-free and I had an idea. I wrote jokes, I hired a director and my show even had a narrative, a 'message'. *Asylum Speaker* was a hit.

Steve Coogan came to see it one night and afterwards, at a party, told me, 'It was the best show I've seen this festival … actually, no, Count Arthur Strong was the best show I have seen. Yours is second best. I think.'

I grinned, my heart soaring. I moved quickly away before he remembered another show he had seen which might put me third.

Comedy agent Addison Cresswell, who is no longer with us, looked after some of the biggest names in stand-up. He was old school and was *the* agent you wanted representing you. I doubt there will be a showbiz agent like him ever again. I hyperfocused on how to get him to be my agent. This was the closest to a plan I'd ever had. I worked hard, smashed every gig and was asked to do a recording for the Paramount Comedy channel. When I came off stage, Addison grabbed me, waggled his finger in my face and announced, 'YOU'RE THE BEST FEMALE COMEDIAN SINCE JO BRAND' and became my manager. Now we were cooking! I was on TV; I was making money. I was also suffering bulimia relapses and I didn't understand why. I was still clueless about ADHD and the connection to my bulimia. I still had no idea I had to look after myself and my mental health, and I was completely overwhelmed. *Move, move, move! Go, go, go!* insisted my internal motor. *Don't think! Just GO!* A huge production company was interested in nurturing a sitcom for me but my head was scrambled and my focus short-circuited. I sat in the meetings, unable to absorb what the producers were saying. I felt totally disconnected.

I worked with Rob Beckett at a gig in Norway once, years ago, and was really struck by how he was taking his increasing fame in his stride. I listened to Rob on a podcast in lockdown. He said that when he decided to stay in this industry and do well, he knew he had to be sure to look after his mental health to cope with all the bad bits – 'So I bought ALL of Ruby Wax's mental health books and read 'em.' This blew my mind. To have the awareness to think: *I'm going to go for this career, so I am also going to take time to get my head right.*

He was a million miles ahead of me. In my day, you just drank until some kind of career happened or you died.

Some kind of career was definitely happening for me. I did *The Secret Policeman's Ball* and smashed it, then I got *Live at the Apollo*. I was on all the chat shows, my tour dates were selling out and I got a book deal. Everyone thought I was on my way to becoming a household name. I married Christian and had a baby boy. Then, my marriage collapsed.

I did not know I had ADHD; my husband did not know I had ADHD. My inability to regulate my emotions made our break-up a million times more painful than it should have been. Now that I understand ADHD and have therapy, now I have worked on rebuilding my self-esteem, there is no way that a man leaving me would be such a devastating catastrophe. Then, however, I felt as though I had been picked up and hurled off a cliff.

I wasn't just sad; I was having a breakdown. But my energy was through the roof. I did not stop for a breath. I drank heavily and absolutely closed the door to any suggestion of taking time off work. Surely all these opportunities would go away if I did? So I went on *The Jonathan Ross Show* when I was still weeping about my ex in public; I did a tour where I just drank on stage and talked nonsense. I said yes to doing *Live at the Apollo* again even though I knew my new material was in no way strong enough. Not only was I crushed by nerves, with material that was cobbled together, I got into a muddle with the stop clock on the stage and overran by ten whole minutes. A crime in television. Everyone, including the producers, could see that I was an utter shambles. I absolutely should not have been working, for at least a few months.

I had a gig in Yorkshire the day after the terrible *Live at the Apollo* gig. I found a field to sit in. I hoped the ground would open and swallow me up because after such a big disaster, it felt like there was no place for me in the world anymore. The ground remained uncooperatively sealed. I called Addison. He sounded exasperated. 'You've let your personal life really affect your work,' he told me. 'I love you; you wear your heart on your sleeve, but I'll be honest with you, I get a headache these days when I mention your name to producers.' Not long after that, he said he couldn't get me anymore TV work. The interest was gone.

Not only had I blown *Live at the Apollo*, I'd also ditched the sitcom opportunity to 'work on my marriage'. I had messed up a lot of jobs by being ill-prepared, or just crying a lot in front of everyone.

I read Rylan Clark's autobiography recently. He talked about his husband leaving him, and how it broke him. It sounded like he was in a similar place to me. He handled it very differently, though. He cleared the decks of any work. For months he just took care of his mental health, away from show business. I could have done that. My family and friends had begged me to do the same. A friend of mine who lived in Thailand said, 'Come and stay with me until you are better.' But I didn't. I ploughed on, crying in TV studios and wailing to anybody who was near me.

Now that I *do* know I have ADHD and have ways to treat it, I can see all the opportunities I missed because I just shut my eyes and ran at them, without preparation and without getting my head right. Addison had done all he could. He'd got me on the panel show *8 Out of 10 Cats*, hosted by Jimmy Carr. All my focus was on my disintegrating marriage. I gave the show no thought whatsoever. I was too locked into anxiety. I could watch stand-up, but watching a TV show I was about to go on felt too much like homework. And, as we know, I don't do homework. My brain went *Homework? Nahhhhhh! We're not doing that! Eat this cake instead. Aww, now you're gonna look fat on TV: better throw it up. And now you're drained and disappointed. What's the point of you trying to do well? You never do well. There is NO room for you in TV. Oh, I know! Drink wine!*

I lost the thread of what was going on whilst on TV. My brain went dancing off somewhere else. When Jimmy Carr came to me with 'What do you think, Shappi?' I had no clue what they had been talking about. I had drifted off. I did *The Chase* without understanding the rules. Same with *Pointless Celebrities*. (Post-diagnosis, I did appear on *Pointless Celebrities* and won!)

I was told about a male comedian who had also not done so well on *Live at the Apollo*. The comic, rightly, felt entitled to ask for a second shot, to make it better: it was granted and he was respected for that. The very idea that I might open my mouth and say, 'Yeah, we need to do that again, I messed up' *on a TV show* sent my brain chemicals shrieking. It was just like when I messed up my French GCSE exam all those years ago, when I was sick on my exam paper and had to go home. I didn't value myself enough to take the exam again. I could have just asked to retake it, but I did not know I was entitled to a second chance. I just sat in a field and self-flagellated. Nowadays, if I am booked for a TV show, I prepare. I go for a run beforehand, I breathe, I take my ADHD medication and I take enjoying myself on the shows seriously. As a viewer, it's no fun watching somebody who is not having an absolute ball. But before my diagnosis, I clung on to my seat, my face fixed frozen, just like the times I have been bonkers enough to get on a roller coaster, with no control.

In 2017, I agreed to appear in reality TV show *I'm a Celebrity ... Get Me Out Of Here!* and got on a plane to Australia *without ever having watched it.*

The producers were very keen for me to do it. I had turned it down several times but for the 2017 show they kept popping up in my life like meerkats, being adorably pushy, even standing in the queue at my book signing at the Edinburgh Festival saying 'please' very prettily.

I don't know why they particularly wanted me that year. I definitely think they had no idea how terrifying 'tabloids-are-interested-in-you' fame was to me. It did not seem like it made your world friendlier. I eventually agreed when they offered me more than what I'd normally make in a year.

I didn't even do the very minimal amount of research and preparation by watching the show. Every time I thought about it, my brain whizzed in another direction. *NO! THAT'S HOMEWORK!*

It was naked fear, I have no doubt. It's a terrifying show. Like with everything else, I just shut my eyes and jumped in without a thought. In this case, literally. 'You're going to jump out of a helicopter, into the jungle', I was told cheerily. I was above the clouds with a camera in my face, strapped to a man who I had just met and who was about to hurl himself, and me, out of the door. I am terrified of heights. I can't look down when I'm standing on a chair, yet here I was, thousands of feet in the air, suddenly hurtling down head-first towards the ground, landing in a lake. The ultimate shock to my system.

At first, you drop head first like a stone. I squeezed my eyes shut and screamed, until the nice man I was strapped to like a giant baby pulled open the parachute. Then we spun around, shooting straight back up in the air, then eventually came the peaceful glide down. All I thought about during the deeply unnatural, surreal and beautiful experience of being in the sky and not being in an aircraft (which is very natural) was how little I see of my friends because of my work, how much I love my life outside of work and how I needed to clear the decks and have a life outside of comedy.

In the *I'm a Celebrity* jungle, I saw close up what it takes to be a reality TV star. It was pretty clear, straight away, that I had a better chance transforming into a gecko. Whether you are talking to someone about their divorce, or announcing that you are going to the toilet, you have to perform what you are saying. 'Guys! I'm going to the loo, right, and I need to talk about how scared I am of spiders because if there's a spider in the dunny, I swear to you guys, hand on heart, I can't lie, I will run out screaming and I don't even care if I've pulled my pants up or not. Honestly.' Then that's the cue for everyone else to shriek and shout how they feel about spiders. 'Oh my God! That is SO what I would do! Honestly, if I even *see* a spider, like, even the thought, I'm like "Oh my God!" I can't even.' Then the camp He-Man would square up to an imaginary spider and say, 'It's alright, I'll go and look and get rid of any in there,' and the others would go, 'Oh my God, you're amazing, genuinely I can't even lie, you're just totally amazing.'

This would go on and on and I would sit thinking, *Just go for your piss* which doesn't make for interesting TV.

The performative empathy of reality TV was fascinating. If someone said they really missed cheese and onion crisps, everyone dropped everything and went to them to hold them in a group hug and to tell them to 'be strong' as though we were tourists kidnapped by pirates rather than professional attention seekers being paid a fortune for camping in a forest for a couple of weeks. Being in that show was utterly bananas. To be shut out of your life, unable to make any contact with anyone who loves you, is surreal. I missed my children to the point of madness and that stopped me being able to have any fun. Also, there were a few loud and intimidating people in there who made it no fun. I was determined not to cry or argue with anyone. I stayed quiet and compliant and happily took all my clothes off when I showered in the waterfall, knowing that MIDDLE-AGED WOMAN GETS HER BAPS OUT would not be tabloid-worthy. If you are not familiar with *I'm a Celebrity*, the viewers vote for who they want to stay in the show each week. If you are not already a national treasure, you have to give the producers something to make you a 'story', something that will either divide opinion or make you a hero. My friend Iain Lee did a genius, very bold thing of eating all of the strawberries which were meant for the whole camp. Easily the biggest story of my series (I know, someone eating strawberries being on the front pages of tabloids and dividing the nation for weeks *is* completely bonkers, but that's reality TV for you).

Iain went from being camp outcast to being one of the three finalists. I just sat politely on a log and was voted out first to have a nice holiday with my children on Australia's Gold Coast. The genuine hunger in the camp took me by surprise.

Having never seen it before, I thought the meals you won were ready-made, like a nice big jacket potato and beans or a hearty plate of spag bol. But no. You won things like a raw quail which you had to chop up and cook with vegetables no one had ever heard of. I became a vegan four months before the show started and I didn't have to eat weird meat. I preferred the rice and beans and just couldn't get excited about 'Whoopie! You won a star! Now chop up this goat with a blunt knife!'

You can't fly straight back to the UK when you come out; your family joins you and you all have to stay at a luxury hotel until everyone is out. The sooner you leave, the longer the holiday you get with your loved ones is. It wasn't just the money that made me agree to it. Addison had died suddenly three years earlier. It was a huge shock. I felt rudderless, treading water. I was older now, with another child, a single mum of two, I was no longer one of the 'bright young things' and had not bitten at the chances I had had to become more established. I had blamed my marriage break-up for that. I didn't know that my unmanaged ADHD, and the anxiety that came with it, had been distorting my idea of what I actually wanted. I had thought that 'success' would bring me some peace, but as I sat in the jungle, drying my pants on a stick over a fire on national television, I just thought, *Why have I been so scared? Why do I feel that every single job I get, every gig I do, is an audition? Why am I waiting to enjoy myself? What am I waiting for? It's all happening right now! My friends, my family, my job: they are all brilliant and happening now! So what the fuck am I doing drying my pants in a jungle?*

Of all the messages I got from people when I got out, the most astute and comforting was from Richard Osman, who understands the medium of television perhaps more than anyone. 'Going into the jungle was your (very clever) way of shocking your system and finding out what's important to you', he wrote. 'In 2018, you will be able to act on what you learned.'

He was right. This kind of fame was not for me. I wasn't good at it and knew it would bring me no joy. Like so many other times in my life, I had to take myself to the very edge to be sure about what I wanted.

I had myriad unhealed emotional wounds, mixed with ADHD chemical deficiencies that made processing them hard. I had thought that once I was famous, I would be cured of anxiety. I was desperate to be cured of it. It robbed me of sleep. It triggered endless paranoid thoughts: *Nobody likes you. You shouldn't have said that, you shouldn't have done that. Everybody is annoyed with you.* I thought that if I was famous, this anxiety would disintegrate. I would have proved myself.

But when I began to get breaks on TV, the anxiety did not go away: it grew. The initial excitement of being booked for a TV show would be dulled quickly. When I came back from *I'm a Celebrity*, I was really famous for about a week. I got mobbed by school kids in Pets at Home. It was the kind of 'fame' that made you hide behind big sacks of sawdust; not the kind I'd dreamed of as a kid. If you want reality TV fame, you have to constantly work to keep yourself in the spotlight, keep your status at the top. Be on the 'right' shows, be seen with the 'right' people and get a professional to do your Instagram. You really have to be a swot to do all this. I've seen how hard people work at fame. They tailor their social media photos. They crop out those whose brand will not serve them. I myself have done this (so sorry, open-spot comics) and have had it done to me (Peter Andre is dead to me). New people, just as talented and tenacious as you, want what you have. So you have to be utterly focused on being the best you can be. There is no wandering off to look for something in a skip to upcycle.

I was not 'fixed' by being on TV. I was even nominated for a British Comedy Award, so why did negative thoughts still shake me awake at night? *It must be because I am not 'there' yet, right? I'm not famous enough yet, so I have to keep climbing.* Life-wasting nonsense.

I spoke to my friend, the brilliant comedian Jen Brister, about this. How I was frantically climbing, thinking I couldn't be happy until I'd reached the top.

Jen, whose career has rocketed in recent years, sipped her tea and shook her head, laughing. 'What did you think is up there? It's dust. It's just dust!'

I'm a Celebrity made me finally understand that no external validation was going to bring me a peaceful head. I still didn't know I had ADHD when I was on the show. But I understood by then that my anxiety was not going to go away because a journalist who thrust a microphone in my face was interested in where I got my shoes.

My vision of success, of what I wanted, was distorted. I had been trying to construct a career in one of the most competitive industries, where you are the product you are selling, when I was emotionally red raw, with no tools or armour to protect myself. ADHD didn't let me think, didn't let me acknowledge what I needed. It just went, *RUUUUU-UNNNNNNNN!!! GO GO GO, YOU IDIOT. WHAT'S THE MATTER WITH YOU?*

I gave very crucial decisions to other people to make for me. In my career and in my relationships. 'Sure! You know best! I mean, I'd rather *not* put pins in my eyes, but what do I know! I'm an idiot! I get everything wrong! Move in!'

But I'm not an idiot and I'm not incompetent. I just don't have a linear thought process. I am not systematic; it's not how my brain works, and it took me a long time to acknowledge my own feelings and feel deserving of asking for what I need. I needed time, I needed rest, I needed therapy. I tried for so long to do things the way other people did them and it just meant I ended up feeling a failure, again and again.

The confidence and self-awareness I have now mean I choose work that I know will be fun. When I am booked for TV shows I prepare, I get my head in the right place and then I thoroughly enjoy them. I remind myself it is not a maths GCSE and I was not booked by accident.

These days, I'm sure if I was asked to do a reality TV show again, I would be in. But this time I'd have a marvellous time taking the piss instead of being polite and I would definitely eat all the strawberries.

LOSING MY SHIT

People with ADHD often have emotional reactions above and beyond what may be considered appropriate. As I imagine you will have picked up on by now, this is something I am quite familiar with.

Your printer doesn't work and instead of troubleshooting, you have a panic attack, is one example I have personally experienced. Having to blink back tears because the air steward misses you out when handing out teas and coffees is another. When a partner mentions, 'Oh, yes I *have* been to the Isle of Wight before, my ex-girlfriend's grandparents are from Ryde,' and you suddenly scream, 'WHY DON'T YOU FUCK OFF TO RYDE THEN? GO AND MARRY YOUR FUCKING EX AND LIVE IN THE ISLE OF FUCKING WIGHT? YOU CLEARLY DON'T LOVE ME!' and sob all night, is yet another.

Of course, losing your shit over seemingly small things isn't all down to ADHD, even if you have ADHD. But ADHD does like to stop you from getting things in perspective. Hyperventilating and sobbing uncontrollably as you scream at your poor family to help you find your shoe with the urgency of someone who is on fire might seem like an overreaction, but in that moment, you can't help but see the lost shoe as a symbol of a lifetime of frustration. You are late for something important – perhaps you are catching a train – and you cannot rely on a simple thing like your footwear present-ing itself to you. You are an idiot, your shoe is an idiot, your life is an idiot and you become engulfed with panic and rage.

This emotional overload is, of course, not about the shoe. There is a build up to it, one which you have not learned to look out for and so cannot put the brakes on and address before you erupt and exhaust yourself. I need to talk about dogs for a moment. It might seem like I am having an ADHD 'moment' (Let's face it, there are plenty of those in this book) and going off on a tangent about dogs but stay with me. It will make sense.

I think all dogs have ADHD. If you are familiar with dogs, you will know how impulsive they are and how you, as their owner, need to anticipate the impulsive, frantic behaviour to help them stay calm. Telling them off doesn't work. My golden retriever, Taylor, barks at other dogs when she is on the way to the park and still on the lead. She is never like this on the way back. All the fun is in the park and she can't wait to get there. The excitement gets too much for her, then 'RUFF RUFF RUFF!' she will go at another dog. It looks scary if you don't know dogs. So I pre-empt Taylor's behaviour. I play with her in the house to get some of the excitement out before we go on the walk, so the fun doesn't start only at the park. We have already had lots of fun, so the walk is calmer. I keep treats in my hand to distract her. If I see another dog coming, we go to the side of the pavement and I get her fully focused on me and the treats.

I have learned a lot about myself through training Taylor. I'd get overexcited too: I would bound up to people who were deep in conversation with someone else and interrupt them. The human version of 'RUFF RUFF RUFF'!

Dogs can be calm one minute and go ballistic the next. A rescue dog I had from Romania, called Benji, was the sweetest, most gentle dog, until one day my teenage son came down the stairs dressed as Elton John. (Having two minutes to dress up as a famous person was a lockdown game of ours.) My son wore my long vintage 1970s coat, with a huge fake fur collar, a hat and my Dame Edna sunglasses. The dog froze with aggression, curled back on his haunches ready to attack and barked wildly and aggressively at my son, who he had never had a problem with before.

Because he was a rescue dog, we hadn't known what his triggers were. Now we discovered that at some point in his life in Romania he had had a terrifying encounter with someone in a long coat or wearing dark glasses, or maybe Elton John himself.

Like Benji, I had triggers but I didn't know what they were or indeed that I had them. My freak-outs seemed to come from nowhere – though that was never actually the case. The build-up would start: tiredness, worry, insecurity about something that I wasn't addressing … then suddenly, WHOOSH! I was a grown woman having a meltdown because I couldn't find a hairbrush. When I was finally calm, an avalanche of shame poured into me again. I could not explain to my loved ones what happened to me because I didn't understand it myself.

It was clear from when I was very young that I didn't even know you *could* process emotions. I had epic tantrums as a child. My brother Peyvand and I both did, but very differently. Mine were fits of crying and screaming and his were running around maniacally like a hyper baboon. His teachers were always calling my parents to discuss his Tarzan impressions and his baboon episodes. Peyvand would go nuts: he'd jump about, shrieking, being really annoying, and there was no controlling him. He was like a noisy rubber ball. He ran away when we were on holiday once and my poor mum feared he'd fallen into a canal. He was found soon enough but she remained grey for the rest of our trip.

Now that I am raising children, I can see sometimes that tears and tantrums are just emotions and frustrations too huge for their tiny little bodies to hold, so they *will* chuck their yoghurt on the floor and turn purple with yelling if they feel they are not being understood. With my children it stopped once they had enough words to say what they needed. (In my son's case, 'Stop that noise'. His first full sentence. I had been singing him a lullaby.) But my tantrums went on until I got help for ADHD in my forties.

I feel protective of my parents when talking about how they missed that my dramatic reactions to things may have been a chemical deficiency, or just the tip of the iceberg on top of a backlog of unprocessed emotions. I don't blame them for a single thing, and I am trusting you not to judge as I tell you about them. Even aside from the trauma of being exiled after the Iranian Revolution, losing everything, being separated from family and having to start from scratch in a new country with a new language, this was after all, the 1970s and 1980s. As a country, we were only just beginning to wake up to the mistreatment of children. Corporal punishment only became illegal in state schools a year before I started junior school. We had only just come round to the fact that thrashing kids for forgetting their sharpener may not be in that child's best interests (private schools only stopped this barbarism in the late 1990s). TV presenter Esther Ranzten helped set up Childline and child abuse was finally something people felt able to talk about out loud. But this was as far as we had got with child welfare.

My parents loved me; they didn't hit me; they did their best to take care of me, so these tantrums of mine were because I was 'bad-tempered' and 'dramatic'. Life at home could be pretty turbulent, though, and 'she's got a short temper like her father' was something I heard a lot. This may be true. But why did my father lose his temper? Trauma has been scientifically proven to be hereditary and scientists believe ADHD also has hereditary elements to it. Perhaps my father and I were both short-tempered not because it is hereditary, like our strong noses, but because neither of us knew what we needed to address to stay calm. We carried on until we blew.

Again, back then, it was unthinkable to imagine there was anything 'wrong' with your child. Looking for neuro-logical differences wasn't an option for most parents in the 1970s and 1980s. Mental health issues carried stigma. There were a few suicides of the sons of family friends as I was growing up and there would be whispers of 'he was mentally unwell', as though this meant taking his own life was inevitable, a reasonable explanation. So even though my mum could see my behaviour wasn't in my own hands, she didn't imagine – or couldn't accept – this was a neurological problem, especially as my behaviour at school was impeccable.

The thinking was that if there *was* something wrong, it would be wrong *all* the time, right? So my temper tantrums must have been wilful. Long into my adulthood I would become frustrated, shout and scream at my family, and they would say, 'How come you don't behave this way outside the house? Why do you let people walk all over you but at home you are so aggressive?' They got angry with me, as though I was deliberately being horrible to them, not understanding that I was desperately masking ADHD outside of the home to appear 'normal'.

I didn't understand either. People with undiagnosed ADHD don't even realise they are hiding something. Without being aware of it, we often hyperfocus on behaving beautifully outside of the home. We bottle up all the pain and frustration, and it all comes out once we are with people we feel safe to unleash it on. I absolutely didn't trust myself not to lose it and make a scene if I acknowledged how I was feeling, so ADHD left me with two settings: utterly compliant and never standing up for myself, or the Incredible Hulk. Nothing in between.

There's an expression in my native Farsi – *asabesh khoordeh*. It means 'Their nerves are crushed.' (I say 'their' because there are no pronouns in Farsi.) I would hear my mum whisper this about me, concerned. She was right, to a point, but the underlying issue was that ADHD short-circuited my executive functions that regulate my emotions. In other words, because of the way my brain is wired, it was pretty much impossible for me to learn to deal with negative emotions and situations in a calm or logical way. Which was particularly unhelpful as, through no fault of my parents', there was often a lot to deal with at home. I know that my mother attributed a great deal of my shattered nerves, the crying and the tantrums, to what I witnessed at home from my dad and the impact of being refugees from a country in utter turmoil.

Early childhood trauma can also contribute to ADHD-type symptoms. My father lost his father when he was just six years old and was sent away to the city, to live in a children's home. Although my grandmother could recite the poets Rumi, Hafiz, Ferdowsi and dozens of couplets off by heart, she could not read and write, which is common for country folk of her generation. So with his dad gone, a school in the city meant my father would be educated. My father once told me that he was 14 before he realised it wasn't normal to be woken up each morning by your own sobs. *I had an extremely sad childhood. I was never allowed to grieve my father. This is affecting my own abilities as a father, so I shall take myself to therapy and begin to heal* was not a thought process open to many people of my father's generation. 'Bury it deep and move on!' was more the way.

My father was a well-known poet and writer by the time he was in his early twenties. After the 1979 revolution, Iran became the Islamic Republic of Iran, with Ayatollah Khomeini as its Supreme Leader. Dissidents in politics and in the arts, like my father, were arrested or executed. My dad managed to flee to London. He continued his writing in exile, publishing a satirical magazine which became very popular amongst the Iranian diaspora now scattered around the globe.

But terror followed us here. As a young child, I sometimes picked up the phone to a horrible voice. 'Your father is scum. Tell him he is going to die.' Then – *click* – they would hang up. Sometimes the calls were even worse. I was around 15 when I picked up the phone and a man quoted our home address to me (which my father had helpfully printed on each page of his magazine, along with our phone number) then said, 'We are going to come and cut off your daddy's head. We are going to rape you and your whore mum.' I dropped the phone and shook with fear. Terror, real terror, feels like you are suddenly filled with a mass of air but somehow cannot breath. It is a hollow, vast, quiet panic. I was alone in the house and struggled to keep my fingers still as I dialled 999.

My father's way of dealing with this sort of thing was to take the piss, make us laugh, make light of the situation. 'Hahaha, we are all laughing! We are all okay!' Even though it felt to me like at any moment men were going to rush into our house and cut our heads off, our unspoken family agreement was to pretend we were not scared.

So my father was very calm about terrorist threats, but he would, intermittently, blow his top to terrifying levels, bellowing and ranting suddenly if we forgot to do something he'd asked us to do, left our toys in the hall or he couldn't find a comb. There was no consistency to the episodes or the thing that would send him over the edge. Sometimes, if he asked you to bring him a pen, and you couldn't find one, he'd be fine. He'd find one himself. Another time, if you couldn't find one, he would rant and rave and make everyone's life hell for hours.

It was like living with an active volcano. Most of the time it was peaceful and pleasant, but after a while it would erupt and shatter everything in its path, including you. The warnings would come: they were quiet, but still there. You knew it was going to blow but you had nowhere to hide.

My father's temper tantrums, like my own, were typical of someone with emotional dysregulation. It is like a switch is flicked. We become different people. He and my mother had epic rows. Loud, unrelenting fights that went on for hours and hours. These did indeed 'crush my nerves'. There was never physical violence (thank goodness, because my mum could have pummelled my father into the ground). But their insults and, later, hiccupping sobs, left us kids shaken to the core. Adults stomping, bellowing, with arms flailing, is petrifying for children. You don't understand why they are not protecting you. I felt hated when my father was angry. It can be devastating for a child when this kind of behaviour becomes 'normal'.

I understand it now, though. Anxiety built up in him; he overloaded himself. He made himself available to every single fellow exile, fan, neighbour who wanted his company, advice or help. Anyone could get his magazine and see our phone number on the back. One morning, a stranger called – a fan of my father's – and said 'I am going to kill myself and I want to meet Hadi Khorsandi before I die.' My father chatted calmly to him for a while, took down his address (it was all the way over in Oxford) and even spoke to the man's wife, who was desperately worried about her husband. 'We have two children', she said. 'They're only eight and nine.'

Peyvand and I were the same age. 'Come on everyone!' my father sang cheerily as soon as he put the phone down. 'Get in the car. We are going to Oxford.' Peyvand and I spent a pleasant afternoon playing with the man's children. They had a stream at the end of their garden with frogs. Utterly mesmerising to two kids from London. The man's wife made everybody lunch, he and my father spoke, and in the evening, we drove home again. The man did not kill himself.

This kind of thing was typical of my father. He would drop everything and run if anyone called for his help, which they frequently did. He did not rest. He overloaded himself and then he would suddenly yell, 'YOU DIDN'T TELL ME MR SHEKARI CALLED LAST NIGHT!' and off he would go into a rage, like a demented silverback gorilla, until he exhausted himself quiet again.

Like me, my father made tight friendships very quickly and, also like me, these friendships were often short-lived. One minute someone was in the very bosom of our family, sharing every little detail with us; the next, we never saw them again. We were both easily hurt and always onto the new, always chasing that dopamine hit.

I wasn't popular like my father. People were always desperate to see him, to talk to him. He was the life and soul wherever he went and I often felt that was how I was meant to be too. It pained me that I wasn't. Emotional self-reliance was not a concept I had heard of or imagined was possible. If a friend didn't call me back straight away, I would obsess about it, call them again and again, leaving increasingly frantic messages with fake chirpiness. But the kind of people who did call back were not the ones I was drawn to. I read 'level-headed' and 'reliable' as 'boring'. I had friends who disrespected and undermined me but were 'FUN!' and this became normal. In my teens and twenties, I made 'die-for-you' best friends and needed them to give me their entire focus, otherwise it felt like my world was falling apart. Jesus Christ, that's asking a little too much of someone you have been out clubbing with a couple of times.

In my teens I clung to a friend I made at college. (Remember Suze, who made me revise for my A levels?) We were best friends, we had a great laugh together, but I was possessive to the point that once we went to university, she ditched me. A bit of an overreaction to me turning up to her and her boyfriend's first anniversary dinner – after all, I did offer to go home afterwards rather than sleep over at theirs.

I didn't understand how to give people space, how to respect boundaries. And I would blurt out hurtful things without thinking. A girl I knew at university was distraught because her boyfriend had left her and was going out with a housemate of mine. In the pub, I said to my usurped friend,

'You think *you've* got problems? *I* have to hear him having sex with Kate every night! They are SO loud.'

It was also fair to say, I had absolutely no chill. When I finally began to have boyfriends, I transferred all this suffocating hyperfocus on to them. If it was ever the other way round, if a friend or a boyfriend was needy with me, I would all but change my identity and move to Honolulu. *That* way around was utterly unacceptable to me. I could not cope with anyone needing *me*. Trying to have relationships without any knowledge that I had ADHD and how it impacted me was like trying to climb a mountain wearing just flip-flops and a sombrero. Doomed to fail and inevitably painful.

An absolute inability to walk away from boyfriends who blew hot and cold wasn't all down to ADHD, but it certainly stopped me from taking a step back and looking at the affect the relationship was having on me. It was like being in a tornado: you know it's destructive but you cling on to the hope that calm will come. One boyfriend had tried to be sensible and put the brakes on a little because 'things are going way too fast' (I asked him to move in with me the third time we saw each other). I said, 'OK, then,' and while he put the brakes on, I called and texted him ten times a day. He would respond with a picture of The Fonz.

I saw a few guys in my twenties, short-lived flings, none satisfactory, and I never thought about whether or not they were what I needed. Some of these men I had no connection with and it left me feeling useless and empty. How *did* people connect with guys? How did some girls just chat to them normally? I either babbled non-stop or was utterly, eerily silent. As for one-night stands, it was almost as though the snap don't-think-about-the-consequences decision to go home with a guy, who did not care about me one bit, was not the path to true romance.

I finally met Don, someone I truly adored, in my twenties. I was a life model at an art college in east London, where he was an informal tutor, using the place as a studio to do his own work. I was 23 and living in a bedsit. He was 37 and living with his mum in the council house he was born in. He was a proper cockney, East End born and bred. He had never been abroad and rolled cigarettes in liquorice papers. He was beautiful, kind, and very, very funny. I found him exotic and intoxicating. He knew everything about the Second World War, Dickens, Leonard Cohen and Bob Dylan. I loved him with all my heart. I was ridiculously shy around him for a long time and had to be pretty bladdered to be able to talk to him. He was skint. More skint than me. I did cleaning jobs and life modelling; he was on the dole and looked after his elderly, bed-bound mum.

I didn't see it at the time, but a great deal of our relationship was him looking after me. I was really bad with bulimia and binge-drinking while I was with Don. He did a lot of mopping up after me with no judgement, while never, ever addressing what I was doing. He came to all my open-spot comedy gigs in grotty pub back rooms across London and, when I didn't have a gig, Don and I usually just sat in my bedsit and drank. We never *did* anything together. The two of us would drink when we woke up in the morning and carry on throughout the day. One day, I insisted we went out to Camden. It was a big deal. But I struggled to get it together to leave the house. This happened to me a lot. When I tried to sort myself out so I could get out of the door and go somewhere, it was like one of those dreams where you are trying to run but can't really move. I would find a shoe, put it down, find another, look for a hairbrush, decide I *had* to take my nail varnish off and stop to have toast. In this way, time ticked on and on and the day moved forward without me, filling me with stress as I tried and failed to get my shit together and get out the door. I was missing the day in Camden I'd been so excited about. It was only down the road. We could walk there. But I'd got into a tailspin trying to get ready to leave. I was crying, screaming and shouting at Don, throwing stuff around the room in frustration because I just couldn't focus enough to organise myself to carry out the simple task of getting out of the door, a crucial component of any day out.

When we were finally out, in the fresh air, walking down my road in Tufnell Park, I was exhausted from my tantrum, my chest still spasming. I was quiet and full of shame. 'Have I spoiled our day?' I asked Don.

'No', he said, putting his arm around me. He gave me a squeeze and kissed the top of my head. 'But you gave it a bloody good go.'

Don and I broke up but remained in touch for a long time. I loved our out-of-the-blue phone calls. He loved me when I didn't have a penny to my name, when I was 24 and had no idea what direction to go in. And he loved me when I couldn't organise myself enough to go out for a walk to Camden and was having a Henry VIII-level meltdown. He came to my rescue many a time after our relationship ended, when I was trying to get my career off the ground. He helped me, his married ex-girlfriend, look after my newborn son while I was on stage.

In 2021, I heard that Don had passed away. I needed him very much not to be dead because I hadn't spoken to him for a very long time. But that is not how death works.

Looking back at Don and a couple of my boyfriends in my twenties, I feel I was lucky. I didn't then know how, with less sympathetic men, I would be treated very badly and not realise it was happening until considerable damage was done.

One boyfriend, Sam, showered me with attention, laughed at all my jokes and told me I was the best thing to ever happen to him. Sam was good-looking, confident and cool. I thought I had finally found love, proper love like in the films. We moved in together and he cried, 'because I'm so happy'. But then, he began to subtly criticise me, so subtly it was almost affectionate. 'You're so messy! It's like living with a Womble' became 'You're messy' and then just 'You're a mess'. He began to look for things in the flat that were out of place when he got home – a teaspoon in the sink, a towel that had slipped to the floor, a cardigan on the back of a chair. He would look at this 'mess' and punish me with a mood, not talking to me for hours, sometimes days, until I apologised. He worked away a lot and when he got back, I would brace myself as he inspected the flat.

'I tidied up!' I'd say brightly, slightly frantically, and he would stay quiet until he found something. 'What's this plant?'

'It's a cactus. We don't have any plants and I thought it would be nice. Homely!'

He wouldn't raise his voice; he wouldn't use a tone that anyone could consider in any way unreasonable. He'd say, 'You didn't ask if I wanted a cactus.'

I would be taken aback and at a loss as to why this was an issue. 'I know, but I didn't think you would mind. It's just a plant. I just thought it was nice.'

And he would nod, unsmiling. 'So you weren't *sure* I wouldn't mind, you just *thought* I wouldn't mind.'

'Erm, yeah.'

'So we are in a relationship and you took a unilateral decision about our home without asking me. Is that fair?'

It was completely bewildering. This questioning, his displeasure, would send me into a panic. He loved me, I loved him, and I had done the wrong thing by buying a plant. He wasn't shouting but I could feel my panic rising. I was getting upset, not knowing what answer to give him to stop him being angry with me.

'I don't get it. It's just a PLANT!'

And he would laugh, mockingly, like I was too stupid to understand. 'It is a plant. It's also a decision you made, on your own, about our shared space when we are in a relationship.'

He would not stop until I had crumbled, until I shouted and cried. Then I was in the wrong. 'Do you think shouting is acceptable? Can we work on you being able to have an adult discussion without ending up shouting at me? I think you need to think about what kind of person you want to be. Do you *want* to be the person who gets aggressive and shouts when their partner is trying to talk to them about what's on their mind?'

And then he would ignore me for days. I would turn the whole thing over and over in my head. 'He loves me, he's upset I bought the plant because he wants to feel respected. It was my fault; I shouldn't have got upset. I should have asked him about the cactus. He was being calm; he didn't shout; I'm the one who shouted.'

He would decide when I had suffered enough, then the love would be back: the nose rubs, the pillow talk, the poems. Until it happened again.

This pattern happened again with another man: let's call him Beelzebub. Beelzebub, again, showered me with affection at first, and once he had me, would casually say things to me like 'I usually go out with supermodels, but you make me laugh.' Or 'An ex-girlfriend of mine has moved to Holland. I'm popping over to stay with her this weekend.' I was upset by this and his response was 'Christ, you're so insecure! What's wrong with seeing an old friend of mine? You see your ex-husband all the time. I don't get insecure about that!' I would frantically, uselessly, argue my point that seeing my ex-husband twice a week for the handover of our child was very different to an ex from five years ago getting in touch out of the blue and him immediately going to see her.

There is an addictive element to relationships with people like Beelzebub, who blow hot and cold, who slowly shake your confidence, make you feel that they are a 'prize' and you are lucky to have them.

When someone declares you are the best thing since disposable wax strips, this can be intoxicating to someone who has ADHD, who is an adrenaline vampire. If you feel you have always been 'too much' for people, 'too intense', then along comes someone who seemingly can't get enough of you, it is irresistible. So you let them into your life lock, stock and barrel. But. It is also unsustainable and it is not real love. It took me a very long time to understand that.

Many of us who have ADHD struggle with creating boundaries or respecting other people's. Our impulsiveness leaps over boundaries without a second thought. 'You are mean, but you are also fun! Come in!' This inability to explain feelings calmly, to lay boundaries that keep harmful people out of your life, needs to be addressed in childhood. We all need to know the signs.

In the years after my marriage ended, I was labelled *mental*, *angry* and *unhinged*. I was hurt and upset, yes, but so were many other people who had break-ups. They didn't run after their ex's car, in the rain, in their socks, screaming at them, repeating behaviours which they have proved to themselves, time and time again, do not get the results they want. When people are like this, as I was, it may very well mean their brain chemicals are just not efficient in the way they should be. It could be because of trauma; it could be because of ADHD. Whatever the reason, the person screaming and sobbing cannot help the way they are behaving. This kind of loss of temper and loss of control urgently needs to be addressed. Even though the person who has lost control is in turmoil, the effects of such behaviour can be terrifying and devastating for those around them. 'Sorry, I have ADHD' or 'I was goaded' is not good enough. If you lose your temper to the point of screaming, throwing things or hitting people, get help to start healing. No one should become a victim of someone else's inability to process their emotions.

My brain could not get my husband leaving into perspective. Meeting him and having him tell me he loved me had been my confirmation that I *was* lovable. When he left me, it confirmed that I wasn't.

I spent some proper time being single in my forties and, with the help of my therapist, began to heal festering wounds and build strong self-esteem. The anxiety I carried had made me unable to properly understand that my words and actions could hurt other people. The affect on my friendships and relationships of finding out I have ADHD has been phenomenal. It turns out, I am *very* supportive, thank you very much, and cool, like The Fonz.

If crying is your emotional response to your boss criticising you or to someone in the pub insisting 'Charlie Chaplin *isn't* funny' (this happened to me many times, without ever having seen any of his films), then you may need to look at why that's happening. I'm not saying if you cry when you can't find the remote control, you have ADHD, but you might want to ask yourself why you're reacting in this way, if only for your own peace of mind. If someone is horrible to you, they haven't 'made you cry': you have cried. There is no shame to it. If you are aware of it, you can do something about it, build your armour, learn how to deal with it. It is possible to learn about your own emotional responses and manage them without continuing to process things the same way you did when you were three.

When a small child cries because their banana is broken, I relate to it. It's not about the banana; it's about not being understood, it's about the sheer injustice of being small and not being given the space to express yourself properly. Maybe you are tired, or bored, or are hungry and want a steak and not a stupid banana. Maybe it's about people invalidating the feelings that are overwhelming you, telling you, 'Don't be so silly'. When I see toddlers howling I think, *I hear you, kid, I hear you. Let it out.*

For years, whenever I heard about ADHD it was in the context of being easily bored, not being able to concentrate on homework and occasionally deliberately setting off a fire alarm. But sorting out your emotions needs focus just as much as sorting out your sock drawer does. The chances are that if you have ADHD, you can't focus on how you are feeling. Feeling what you are feeling is one thing but acknowledging your feelings, allowing yourself to have them, letting them flow until they are done, is another thing altogether. When you don't acknowledge them, they build up, get rowdy, then they explode out of you suddenly when you are looking for your purse and your partner, mum or child says, 'Where did you see it last?' ARGGHHH!!!

ADHD can be the great energy drain, exerting itself in useless, resolution-less fighting with partners or anti-vaxxers in the ASDA car park (long story: I was right, he was an idiot, that's all you need to know). Altercations with strangers were fairly regular occurrences for me when I was overloaded and needed to let off steam. I live on a narrow street that some motorists use as a rat run, then get annoyed when we have deliveries or they are stuck behind the bin collection van. *BEEP, BEEP, BEEP* they go, angrily. If I was at home and had a stress build-up, I'd hear those beeps and out into the street I would run. 'He is doing his JOB! Have some patience!' And the already riled motorist, who may well have had ADHD too, would rage at me about the outrageousness of a supermarket delivery van not just hurling the ten bags of groceries on the pavement and speeding off to clear the way for Mr/Ms Purple Face. If they heard me shouting, one of my neighbours would invariably come out to support me (we all get annoyed at the Beep Beep Beep-ers in my street) and I would calm down a bit and stop shouting, because the back-up meant validation and support. Also, *do you really want to risk a brawl in front of the neighbours?* is a thought that does eventually break through.

This part of my behaviour is significant. The problem was always not knowing how wound up I was until it was too late. I have had proper ding-dongs on public transport with people who have shoved me. At a local kids' show, another mum pushed past me rudely as I was consoling my teary daughter in the aisle. *Her* problem, not mine, right? But it was Father's Day and, what with one thing and another, it is a day that can trigger me. I sat next to the woman and quietly wound her up until she threatened to punch me. Clearly Father's Day triggered her, too.

These needless altercations with strangers never happen to me anymore. The need to win an argument, put someone in their place, came from my mind storing up all the times I did *not* stand up for myself. When a bloke tutted at me because I was not going fast enough down a crowded tube platform and I went into aggressive Yorkshire Terrier mode, that was because that old wound was made sore again. And ADHD meant I would react impulsively and immediately, without considering that the bloke I was yapping at might also lose his temper.

THE TRAMPOLINE

I was obsessed with having a baby. I had only been with Christian for six months when I told him 'I WANT A BABY'. I was 32. All the noradrenaline and dopamine that was stimulated when we were together intoxicated me: we call these chemical reactions 'being in love'. I had had some tests done because of pain I was having and the doctor mentioned one of my fallopian tubes may be damaged. My brain whizzed with panic, 'Will this affect my fertility ?', I asked. The doctor said, because of my age, if I wanted to have babies I should start trying and if it doesn't happen, come back and 'we'll see what's what'. This is fair enough advice and probably the same advice given to a lot of women in their early thirties. My brain, however, processed this as a state of emergency. I immediately went home and shrieked, 'We have to start trying for a baby RIGHT NOW,' at the man I had only just started to share a bookshelf with.

'Can't we wait a while?' he asked.

'NO!' I wept. 'I HAVE to start NOW! The doctor SAID.'

I could think of nothing, absolutely nothing, but having a baby. Baby baby baby. I had to be pregnant and although I tried to fix my face into 'I am listening to your needs' mode when my boyfriend tried to talk about it, I did not, for a second, actually hear his needs or feelings. (I know how that makes me sound, by the way. This is not a glory story.) Pleas of 'Can we think about it for a while?' and 'Can we wait for a bit?' sent me into a panic free fall, as though I was in a burning building and I could see the escape route, but someone was tugging on my arm, saying, 'I'm not ready to leave just yet, can't we discuss our options?' I had no method of putting my thoughts and feelings into a logical context. I was driven by this one very urgent desire, need, to get pregnant.

We got married the following year and agreed to start trying after that. I had our son a few days before our first anniversary.

Having a baby, it seemed, required homework in the form of antenatal classes. I went to one class and that was it. I couldn't handle it. It was like being shut up in school again. I fidgeted, at a loss to understand how any of the others could sit still while the woman talked to us without the slightest effort to be entertaining. I didn't expect her to be unicycling around the room juggling grizzly bears, but anything other than a talking pamphlet would have been so welcome. I don't want to be disparaging – though admittedly I am making no clear effort to stop myself – but *come on*! This was about birth! The miracle of life! Yet the antenatal class managed to make it as riveting as a speed awareness course. I couldn't stand it. I went off to get a cup of tea and left all the listening to my husband, who filled me in later about meconium and green poo, which was very useful at 3am on that first night when I was alone with my tiny pink child, chiselling the black goo off his bottom.

I did not buy any baby books. The ones I was given sent me to sleep. I should have read them to the baby.

The people who made a whole project out of having a baby were the same ones who, at school, would do their homework the day it was set. They were a different animal to me, these mothers-to-be who read and planned and learned the biology of what was happening. Who would, no doubt, keep a beautiful book with all the 'firsts' noted down in it. I told people, 'God, I won't be one of *those* mums. I'm actually just going to be present with my baby instead of making a record of every time it farts.' I scoffed, 'My grandmother had nine babies. She didn't go to antenatal classes or read a ton of "how to not kill your baby" books. It's an *industry*. It's *capitalism*.' I was quite an annoying, judgemental arse. But, as with most annoying, judgemental arses, I was projecting, because the truth was, it wasn't that I didn't *want* to be like these other mothers: I *couldn't*.

My anti-capitalist stance didn't seem to affect my buying equipment for the baby. Before my son was even born, he had two cots (one for at home and one at my parents' house), two Moses baskets (in case we lost one at the river?) and an absolute monster, four-wheel drive tank of a pram, which seemed bigger every time I looked at it and sat in the corner of our very tiny flat taking up far more space than was reasonable.

The midwives gave me all sorts of information about breathing and different birthing options. I didn't listen to a word of it. My mind raced past them like Road Runner. My waters broke in the middle of the night. *Dammit.* I recalled

someone with medical qualifications telling me what to do
when this happened, but I couldn't remember what it was. I
woke Christian up; he seemed to be looking to me for a steer
as to what to do. We went back to bed. It all came back to me
when the contractions started. A midwife! Yes, I had to call
one of those. 'Take some paracetamol and go back to bed,'
she said. Then she went back to bed. We were too excited,
though, and also, it turned out that contractions were immo-
bilising and pretty painful.

For some reason, I insisted we got a cab to my parents'
house. Then, when the contractions got really bad, my dad
drove us to hospital. I still can't believe that you can survive
that much pain. Apparently, there are breathing techniques
you can use, but I screamed my way through them because
I didn't stick with the antenatal classes or read any books
to prepare myself.

The one thing the contractions did do was very definitely,
very firmly, put me in the present. The midwife said the
anaesthetist wasn't available. ADHD does not shy away from
a 'scene'. Mine certainly didn't. I'm not saying that you *have*
to have ADHD in order to stomp around in your gown in the
corridors of a hospital, bent double like Quasimodo, bellowing, 'I'M NOT HAVING A FUCKING HIPPY BIRTH! GIVE
ME AN EPIDURAL OR I WILL FUCKING DIE!!! I NEED
AN ANAESTHETIST!' But it probably helps. A nice doctor
called Ahmed appeared very shortly afterwards and stabbed
my spine with delicious drugs. See? Absolutely no need for
antenatal classes.

The moment they put my pretty son in my arms and his gigantic saucer eyes locked into mine is the part I don't just remember – I still feel as if I am there again. It was like he was talking to me. 'Did you SEE what just happened? Did you see it? What the fuck! And are you her? You are my mum, yes? I see. Wow! That was *intense.*'

It's normal, after you have a baby, to have intrusive thoughts. Thoughts that pop into your head with no warning, like *What if a tree falls on the pram?* and *What if I leave him in the bath? I'm going to walk over to his Moses basket and he will be blue and quite dead.* These thoughts flash suddenly in your head and I never shared them with anyone. Because I was supposed to be a perfect picture of motherhood and no one tells you this sort of thing can happen. With my daughter, six years later, the intrusive thoughts lasted for longer. We were at the Melbourne International Comedy Festival when she was almost one, staying on the 40th floor of a hotel, with a balcony. *It would be nice to die with the children* flashed up in my head. I locked the balcony door and sealed it shut with duct tape. Anyone who's experienced thoughts like these, whether they're one-offs or part of a mental health condition like OCD, knows how upsetting they can be. It's important to get the help you need. I told my brother who was in London, who took it quite well actually. He called me every day, several times a day and during the night. 'Tell the people you are with', he encouraged me.

But I found it incredibly hard to tell anyone I wasn't well. I had spent my life masking, being 'Happy Shappi!' (never call me that, by the way), and I didn't want to be seen as not able to cope. In the end, I mumbled to Sara Pascoe, a friend who was also at the festival. She is a kindness machine and an emotional genius. She quietly mobilised the troops and we all went to the beach for the day. For my kids, it was another fun day, but for me, it felt like being rescued.

My grandmother with the nine children called me from Iran. She wasn't interested in the cooing, 'how WONDERFUL' side of new motherhood. She asked kindly and simply, 'Do you love your baby yet? Don't worry if you don't. It will come.'

I DID love Cass, my beautiful boy, but in those first few days I was shell-shocked and in pain. I'd torn during the birth and had had lots of stitches. My midwife told me to get a mirror and have a look at my vagina to 'reconnect with yourself'.

I did. 'How was it?' my husband asked.

'It looks like I've been shot in the twat,' I answered.

Back in 2006, the only thing I knew about postnatal depression was what I had heard about women who sink into bleakness and can't hold their baby or don't feel anything for it. That wasn't me. My son was like my heart living outside of my body. I ached with love, but also with terror. *OH MY GOD HE'S SO DELICATE AND HELPLESS! THE WORLD IS FULL OF CATASTROPHE! PUT HIM BACK IN!*

The intrusive thoughts in most women fade. When sleep returns and the body recovers, anxiety subsides. But ADHD offers free accommodation to intrusive thoughts and for me, it made sure that motherhood was a plug-in to a world of fear. The dark, horrible thoughts stayed in my head and whirred around and around until everything was bleak terror and every news story I had ever read about a child being harmed haunted me. The fact that all over the world, children were being mistreated was the dementing thought that became an obsession. *HOW CAN I BE HAPPY WHEN THERE MAY BE A CHILD IN KUALA LUMPUR WHO IS SAD?* The thoughts repeated in an endless loop. It was hell. I began doomscrolling online, horrible news stories about children, knowing I was just hurting myself more. The unanswerable question of *How could anyone ever hurt a child?* clawed at me and didn't go away. My anxiety was off the scale. We moved into a new house and Cass had his own room. He was a calm little soul and quickly settled, but I would creep in and sleep on the floor in case someone tried to climb in through the window and take him.

A huge news story broke about yet another child who had been murdered by their parents and it dominated the news. When I took my boy to parent and baby classes, I couldn't understand why everyone wasn't talking about it. Why were they all acting normal and not shrieking maniacally at the cruelty of the world and the loss of this beautiful child? It wasn't that I cared more than other parents: it was that I couldn't process this, I couldn't take a step back; the horror engulfed me to an irrational extent. It's normal to be saddened and horrified when you hear that a child has been harmed, but to sob on your own baby all night, too scared to leave him alone for a second, to be plagued by catastrophic images and thoughts – well, that was anxiety on crack.

These repetitive, negative thoughts were not new to me. I'd just never had so much to lose. In the past, they had been anxiety about friendships, family dynamics, my career, my relationships. The thoughts would spin round and round; they would cost me sleep. But now I had a baby. Any harm coming to Cass, or losing him, would be unsurvivable.

On top of everything, of the two cots I had bought, the one at my parents' house was the fancier one. It had little wooden balls in the headboard which the baby could play with. But the one at our home didn't. I obsessed about the fancy cot. 'We need to swap them!' I pleaded to Christian, who did not share my sense of urgency.

I was throwing up a lot again. I had been all through the pregnancy. There was an Overeaters Anonymous meeting very near our new house and I started to go. In the first session I went to, people were sharing stories about abusive relationships, self-harm, suicide attempts. When it was my turn to talk, I said, 'I bought two cots for my baby and THE ONE AT MY MUM'S HOUSE HAS WOODEN BALLS! THE ONE AT MY HOUSE IS PLAIN! I want to swap them but my husband just doesn't understand! He says "A cot's a cot!"' Then I burst into tears while the suicidal man next to me fetched tissues and the woman who self-harmed reached over and gave my hand a supportive squeeze. These people understood me. These people knew that a cot is NOT JUST A FUCKING COT!

Christian did not embrace the whole 'making new parent friends' thing. But now we had moved to a new area and I needed friends. I was as daunted by walking into a parent and toddler group on my own as I would have been going to a nightclub alone when I was 18. *BILLY NO-MATES!* screamed a siren in my head. Jesus! Was I still like this? I had forgotten this social paranoia, thought it was left behind in my youth, but no. It was just that on the comedy circuit, where I had been absolutely entrenched for the last ten years, people were very chatty; they came up to you, and we were always drinking so I'd been hoodwinked into thinking that I was now a socially confident person. But now here I was, in a room full of new mothers, feeling like the kid in the playground on her first day who had wet herself.

As ever, it looked like everyone fitted in except for me. I forced myself to walk over to a small group who were chatting. How did they do this? How did they just gather and start talking about their babies and not be weird? How were they so normal? How did people do this gentle, surface chit-chat?

The group did not immediately acknowledge me. I held my steel until someone caught my eye and I smiled. It probably just looked like wind, so I added a 'hello' and I was in! 'My name's Shappi.' I very nearly added, 'and I'm a compulsive overeater' out of 12-step habit. She said, 'I'm Helen', and introduced the three other woman, whose names I didn't catch because I was in a vortex of 'new social situation' panic and so my ears didn't work.

I was doing okay, though, nodding a lot, smiling. But after just a moment, another woman came in the little church hall and the group warmly welcomed her with hugs and cooed over her very tiny baby with a little tube in his nose.

They all knew her already. *These bloody NCT groups*, I thought to myself. I hadn't joined one and often found myself the odd one out in clusters of them who had all known each other since they were pregnant. I held a rictus grin until someone said, 'Oh, Shappi, this is Caroline. Shappi's new here.'

Caroline gave me a friendly smile. 'It's his first outing! We've only just come out of hospital.' She looked tired and worried and the fuss the other mums made of her told me that Caroline had been through the mill. My heart went out to her and her miniature baby.

Helen politely filled me in. 'Baby Marcus was three months premature.'

Oh lord. I wanted to cry. He was a beautiful little mite. I wanted to hug Caroline and tell her that her baby was a precious little nugget of heaven. However, my brain was in an ADHD scramble of panic. The words that blabbed out of my mouth before I could stop them were, 'Fab! So you got bonus time with your baby!'

The group stared at me. Caroline, bless her, said, 'Er, well, that's one way to look at it.'

I was mortified. It was sheer nerves and inability to take a bloody breath before I reacted which made me say something so massively inappropriate. 'I'm so sorry, I didn't mean to joke …' I began, but it was pointless. They averted their eyes until I walked away. My son, in his sling, looked up at me and smiled, with no idea that his mother had just made us social pariahs.

When Cass was six weeks old, we went to visit my husband's family in Nottingham. I showed off my son, the baby boy I had longed for and was looking after with utmost care and tenderness. It was a beautiful sunny autumn day. The family were all out in the garden. We thought it would be sweet to put the baby down on the trampoline, use it like a giant bouncing chair. I stood over my tiny boy and bounced him ever so gently as his father cooed, 'Is that a smile, baby boy? It's fun, isn't it, my beautiful boy?' My heart filled with love for my baby, my life. I jumped up high, and bellyflopped onto the trampoline, sending him flying. Not that high, but horrific nonetheless.

He went up, then down, and was fine. I was not fine and neither was his father.

'What the FUCK are you doing?' he cried out as he took our boy and examined him.

I did not know what I was doing. I knew that I'd just bellyflopped on a trampoline that my precious newborn son was on but I had no answers as to why. I was sleep deprived, yes, but plenty of new mums are sleep deprived without accidentally catapulting their child into the air.

Looking back, I was somewhat overwhelmed. I had fussed and fretted about our boy's first long car journey. I did not know my husband's family well. I wasn't comfortable making polite small talk and one of his relatives had made a stupid joke which alluded to the fact that my son was mixed race, which I had not called him out on and it had sent me into some disarray. I was masking, bottling emotions that were pinballing around and wouldn't settle. I was in a social situation where anything other than small talk would have been like eating from the buffet using just my face. I was being so careful not to say anything weird like 'he called my baby a camel' and spoil the afternoon.

I shouldn't have been out there. I should have stayed in the front room, with their sweet dogs who slept on the sofa gently farting. I should have sat quietly with them, and my baby, listening to whale music, perhaps also farting gently, avoiding the noise and chatter in the garden. I did not know I needed this. I had no idea that being still and quiet was an option. I am willing to bet, that now I know I have ADHD, no situation would arise where I would put a fucking baby on a trampoline in the first place. I would be able to take a moment to think and would decide, *No. The baby shall remain safe in my arms. I am finding this barbeque too noisy. I'll be inside with the sleeping, trumping dogs.*

There were many reasons that meant my marriage did not survive. My impulsiveness and whirring ADHD brain meant I would change plans at the drop of a hat. I'd come back from a playgroup with a cluster of mums, fill our house up with noise without giving it a second thought, but Christian needed preparation, planning. He would be discombobulated by a sudden change of direction. 'A picnic? But I thought you wanted to go to the zoo?!' It's hard to imagine how any marriage could withstand such chaos. Neither of us understood each other. The different needs of neurodivergent people was information totally unavailable to us at the time. I'm not saying that if we had known about ADHD and 'the spectrum' we would have stayed together. But we would definitely have split up more compassionately.

I was destroyed by our break-up. Not words I use lightly. I was in pieces. Little tiny pieces. Every single morning I felt like a Mr Potato Head toy being hurled at a wall by a freakishly strong toddler. The toddler would batter me to pieces and put me back again all wrong. I'd spend the rest of the day with an arm where my nose should be and ears for my eyes, in utter disarray.

Much like with labour, my ADHD motor drove me ahead with no resources to step back, take a breath and figure out how to navigate this new world I found myself in. My son was just two when Chistian and I separated. I found being in a different room to my baby very hard, so having to let him go to his dad for two nights a week was traumatic. When he was at this new house I assumed my heart would just give out, in the dark of some of those nights. I thought it would probably just stop; explode. How much pain could it hold, after all? Surely it would just pop like an overinflated balloon? There was nothing poetic about my pain; there were no songs to be written. It was just a heavy, agonising weight, dragging me down.

Acting with wisdom and calm made logical sense to me. I tried. But all my inner screaming and crying poured out whenever I spoke to Christian. All my communication with him was a tantrum. 'If you just speak to him calmly, things will be better,' people said, to try to help me. But it was out of my hands. In every interaction with him I reacted with trauma; wounds were endlessly reopened and I was freefalling off a cliff again.

I was at least aware that I needed to talk to someone. Not all therapists know about ADHD, though. My current therapist has ADHD himself and if I had found someone like him, someone who saw that my inability to process my situation, my emotions, with something other than naked rage and panic might be a chemical imbalance, it would have helped. But the therapy I had involved me talking endlessly about my childhood and my relationship with my parents. It might have helped eventually but all took too long. I stopped going to therapy.

There is sadness to deal with, being diagnosed late in life – my education, my needless frustrations, the erosion of my self-esteem – but none of that gets close to the grief I feel for my son in his very early years, when I was so blindsided by my marriage breaking up, so despairing, that he frequently saw me sobbing or shouting or just not being 'present'.

I was on tour at a theatre in Bridgend in Wales. I sat backstage, sobbing and in such pain about the divorce that I sank into blackness. It terrified me. How could I survive this? Though a comfortable thought, ending my life was not an option. I had my beautiful little boy who I couldn't leave and who was a magical, deep-thinking universe of joy.

A dog. I needed a dog. A dog would make my life more bearable when my son was away and it would also give Cass a cheery soul around the place, to offset his heartbroken mother, who cried all the time. I immediately set about finding a puppy and picked it up the next day. Hello, impulsive behaviour!

I had never had a puppy before and so I didn't know how different they are to cats; how insane it is to get one when you are on tour and how they masturbate furiously against the leg of everyone who comes through the front door. Some neighbours called the council and complained about the noise because when I went out, the dog went out of the cat flap and barked in the garden until I returned. I wasn't coping and that wasn't fair on the dog. I think Benji (I DO like to call dogs Benji) the Tibetan Terrier cross is the first dog who 'went to live on a farm' who genuinely did go to live on a farm.

A saviour did come to me eventually in animal form. I had popped into the pet shop to buy fish food and Oscar, a tabby kitten, jumped in my arms and asked me to take him home. Oscar the tabby has never left my side. As I write this, he is curled up on my desk, keeping me company, and, apart from the biting habit he has picked up in his middle age, he is hands down the best ADHD-spontaneous, don't-think-about-the-consequences decision I ever made.

The abundance of energy my ADHD motor gave me, and my pathological spontaneity, did at least make for some glorious times with Cass. 'Are we doing anything today, Mummy?' he asked me one morning when I had loads of work to do, all quite urgent. 'Yes! We are going to Hastings to find a smugglers' cave!' And in ten minutes we were out of the house, going towards the train station. He wheeled his little Paddington Bear suitcase as I quickly booked into a hotel online (which, I discovered when I got there, was next to a place the locals called 'smack alley') and frantically googled 'smugglers Hastings' to find there was indeed a smugglers' cave attraction there.

Sometimes, when it got dark and was very late, I'd say, 'Let's go for a midnight adventure!' and out we would go, me and my little child, our coats over our pyjamas, creeping about our neighbourhood, while I told him all about the elves and pixies which came out when everyone was in bed. When it poured with torrential rain, me and Cass would be the only people out in it, getting soaked to the skin, dancing in and out of puddles.

I took my son everywhere I could with me. My little side-kick. He was such a curious, intelligent, relaxed little chap and made a wonderful travelling companion when I went to comedy festivals abroad. There were constant new friends, movement and bustle. The manic extent to which I needed to be in the thick of things, I have no doubt, was connected with ADHD. I kept nothing of my break-up private. I talked about it constantly to all these new people who I brought into my life. This is something I would not do now. My friendship circle is much smaller. I protect my privacy, lay boundaries, because I am able to process my feelings instead of chucking them in the air like confetti.

Meanwhile, my ferocious inner monologue screamed, *MY SON MUST HAVE AN EXCEPTIONALLY HAPPY CHILD-HOOD!* There is a perfectionism that can come with ADHD that can mean you can't finish a task, because if there is the slightest mistake you start again and wind up endlessly starting from scratch. My perfectionism affected my parenting. I obsessed about Cass having THE BEST TIME POSSIBLE AT ALL TIMES. At Christmas, I dressed as Santa and had all Cass's little friends and their mums over. They shrieked as I dashed about our estate. 'There he is! There he is!' The little girl who was a whole year older than everyone, and a bit too big for her boots if you ask me, declared, 'It's NOT Santa! It's Cass's mummy!' and got a massive snarl from behind my state-of-the-art white beard. If I saw men digging the road, I would dash home, grab him and RUSH out in a wild panic, stressing at him to hurry in case they stopped digging before we got there, in case his childhood was ruined.

We went to Richmond Park to fly his new kite and it got stuck in the highest branches of the most enormous old oak tree. My son was in tears. Getting that kite out of the tree remains, to this day, once of the greatest achievements of my life. It was all wrapped up in my obsession with providing my son with an idyllic childhood despite us becoming a single-parent family. Some would have put more energy into accepting their single-parent status rather than spending a whole afternoon swearing at a tree, but we all travel our paths at our own pace.

Friends and family could see that I was struggling. I cried a lot and was full of anger toward Christian. It's hard for those who love you to know what to do when you are going through something like this. Some listened, endlessly; some still kept telling me to read *Eat, Pray, Love*. 'Honestly!'

they'd gush. 'It's ALL about how to survive heartbreak. It's a survival manual for divorce.' They meant well but I couldn't read someone else's story of survival when I was in the place I was. It was like they were chucking a *How to Swim* book at someone who was in the middle of drowning.

I did listen to my brother. He is wise and very into yoga and meditation but the slowness of these things infuriated me. A deep breath? Who's got the time? Panting like a dog works perfectly well for me. My brother persisted so I went to a local meditation class and found myself thinking, *Lady, hurry this* up! *I've got shit to do!* Which wasn't really the right vibe. I also did no research on the classes I went to. I simply went into a door with a sign outside saying YOGA. At one, a nice woman massaged my feet as I sobbed about my divorce. I paid a fortune for a course of classes and spent a lot of time tapping my solar plexus. I went with it all, thinking, *Well, I do feel more relaxed after coming here.* But then they asked me to go on an away weekend and have a picture of my aura taken. My lack of actual research, my ADHD resistance to any research or planning, had led me to accidentally join a cult.

Five-and-a-half years after I had Cass, I found out I was pregnant again. The father of my baby, let's call him Head-for-the-Hills, was someone I had been in a relationship with but he chose not to stick around when I told him I was pregnant.

He also did not respond well to my endless screaming that he had to be in my child's life. Friends and family kept telling me to stay calm, that I wasn't going to get anywhere by shouting. The idea that I had to behave in a certain way to coax him into fatherhood sent my neurons into a frenzy of *Attack! Attack! We are being attacked!* Why would anyone need coaxing into meeting their flesh and blood; why should I treat him like an alley cat about to skedaddle?

I was 12 weeks pregnant with my daughter when my divorce finally came through. I needed to move nearer to my parents and went into hyperfocus mode. I did not waste any time. The first house I saw was perfect but out of my price range. I borrowed money for the deposit. The day I moved in, I started filming *Celebrity MasterChef.*

Bear with me: I'm going to talk about Rylan Clark again for a moment. It is relevant, I promise. I had never watched Rylan on *The X Factor* or *Celebrity Big Brother.* I knew nothing about him. Then, one day, in the car, I turned on Radio 2 and was blown away by this funny new breath of fresh air with a really strong Essex-via-East End accent and utter self-assurance. His intelligence shone through his humour. Who WAS this radio superstar? Rylan, of course.

He is a career hero of mine because he absolutely demanded a career in show business and didn't let the snobby attitude of a lot of people in the media get him down. His accent, his dazzling veneers, his fake tan and his obsession with reality TV would make most people think he'd be a flash in the pan, but he's gone from being a reality TV contestant to being one of the best-loved TV presenters we have. You simply cannot argue about someone who has the focus and intelligence to harness their talent like he does.

Anyway, like me, he was on *Celebrity MasterChef.* The way he wrote about the experience in his book was fascinating. He took it so seriously. He'd never cooked before and learned. He was a finalist, then became a host judge on further series and went on to present *Ready Steady Cook*. I, however, just saw it as a date in my diary. A massive TV opportunity when I had stopped getting booked for so long, and I didn't take it seriously. I had just got a new house, I was pregnant, and instead of thinking, *Here's my second chance at TV*, I buried my head in the sand and bought a gigantic rabbit hutch and two rabbits.

The longer you stay on *MasterChef*, the more money you get. I knew if I got to the third round, I'd be able to make enough to breathe for a while as I recovered from the C-section.

To be fair, I had cooked goat before. I didn't realise how long it would take and yes, it was mostly raw, and that is not a good thing. I understand that now. Also, yes, in hindsight, putting 5 litres of double cream into an industrial vat of custard powder *did* make yellow cement instead of the desired custard; they were quite right to get annoyed about that and yes, I should have read the label first and yes, I did notice it was very thick milk, but I was up against the clock and in a panic.

They loved the Persian lamb and aubergine dish I made but it was clear I was messing about, and I got booted out in the third round.

Rylan played it very differently from me. He respected the show, the audience and the chance he was given. He respected himself, dammit. Whereas I sabotaged myself by putting all my energies into learning about rabbit care and assembling a flat-pack hutch, which clearly stated it was a two-person job, and not a one pregnant-person job. I should have looked up how to make a roux. Or at least what a roux was. But that would have been doing homework. My ADHD could never do homework.

I made friends with my neighbours on my new street. I introduced myself to the immediate ones when I first moved in, taking round wine and praying they would be nice and not teetotal. Thankfully, they were all lovely boozers. My elderly next-door neighbour was very kind to me, even after I called the police because I had convinced myself she had been murdered.

She hadn't been. The man I saw leaving her house was her son and she had left the back window wide open because she'd been a little warm. When the three police cars came with their blue lights whirling and sirens blaring, I met yet more of my friendly neighbours, who all came out to see what was going on.

One way I have unconsciously managed my ADHD since I was a child has been to find friends in my immediate vicinity who have the skills I massively lack: organisation and practicality. In my new neighbourhood the children all went to the same school, so my new friends told me what was going on there, when to bake (buy) a cake for the bake sale, when the holidays were and frequently, what class they were in.

When the piano I had impulsively bought was plonked on the pavement outside my house, my new neighbours brought it in. I am still hoping that one day I will learn to play it.

I had a C-section with my daughter, Vivie, the day before my fortieth birthday. That first night, I should have been relaxing with my lovely, longed-for little girl, but, against sensible instinct, I called her father, who did not want to talk to me. So then I called *his* father: 'I just want to let you know you have a granddaughter.'

He said, 'I don't like to get involved in my son's relationships.'

That familiar tidal wave of 'loss of control' whooshed through me. I was hysterical. 'We haven't had a tiff! I've had a baby,' is what I was trying to say but it came out more 'WEHAAAAAAN'T HAAAADGHGH ARGH TISHFT AAHVHADABAAAAAYBBA' and then heaving sobs.

As with every relationship, if I had understood my brain better, I would have handled that situation much more calmly than I did. But I felt like I was being hurled out of a window. Repeatedly shrieking 'WHAT KIND OF MAN REFUSES TO SEE HIS CHILD' down the phone until my throat bled a few hours after giving birth bizarrely did not help a very delicate situation.

The night duty nurse, a Nigerian woman called Wendy, came in, saw me crying and said, 'Ah good. Your milk is coming.' She was an angel to me that first night, sitting by my bed and holding my hand, as I howled and wept for my baby girl, fresh into the world and already abandoned by her dad. Wendy sat with me and patted my hand, cutting straight though any niceties or mollycoddling. She told me she raised her children alone. 'And now they are both strong girls, both at university,' she told me. 'You have to be strong too. You have a big job to do.' She then informed me that *Pretty Woman* was on in a minute if I wanted to watch it. I did. Very much.

My brother arrived and Wendy turned a blind eye to the champagne he'd brought. Until he needed help opening it and she popped the cork for him. She took my daughter off for a walk 'so you can just relax'. And I did. I celebrated my fortieth birthday with my brother, healing from major abdominal surgery and enjoying the story of a sex worker who falls in love with an emotionally unavailable man.

My family were constantly with me in the first few weeks of Vivie's life. In the midst of all this recovery and nesting with a new baby, a woman I vaguely knew came to stay for a week as she needed digs in London. There had been a teeny, tiny, sensible voice from a distant part of me that had whispered, *I think this may be too much for you.* But my **people-pleasing,** ADHD brain said, *YES! OF COURSE! NO PROBLEM!*

Not long after, a new young comedian got in touch for advice about his first Edinburgh show. Again, 'It's not a good time, I've just had a baby' came out as, 'Sure, I live in Ealing. Come over to my house. What was your name again?' I sat and breastfed and gave solidly rambling advice about the comedy industry to this chap, who really didn't know where to put himself. Then I handed him my daughter and had a bath.

I don't know how his Edinburgh show went and I still can't remember his name.

My daughter was very different from my son. He had been a calm baby, able to soothe himself easily. Vivie needed to be glued to me at all times. If I even broke eye contact with her, she cried. If I was holding her and chatting to a friend, I had to keep my conversation positive; if my chat went to expressing frustration at my exes or I moaned about the Co-op being out of blueberry muffins, she howled.

When she was five, I decided she needed to meditate. I was so worried that she was like me. So, while we were getting ready for school, I found a kids' meditation channel on the internet and said, 'Let's sit down on the mat and listen.' She did not want to listen; she wanted to run around the room. She is almost ten now and still enjoys acting the scene out in front of people: 'Mummy shouted at me, "SIT DOWN AND MEDITATE! RELAX OR I WILL GET CROSS!"'

Both my children have seen my undignified loss of control, my temper, usually when I was in a rush and couldn't find my keys, and so would lob a book at a wall and call the door a bastard. I'd then cry and apologise for shouting, hold my children, who would say, 'It's the door you should say sorry to' because they had learned to make me laugh as a way of taking care of me. This broke my heart because it came from their relief that they weren't scared anymore. I had frightened them. The 'Scream, Shout, Cry, Say Sorry' parenting style was never covered in any of those baby books I didn't read.

When my son was three, he was, as usual, refusing to put on his shoes to go to nursery. This is normal for a three-year-old.

He didn't have the sense of urgency that I did to keep to time and was giggling his head off as I tried to wedge his little trainers onto his feet. On most other days, I would giggle with him, make a game of it. But on this day, thanks to whatever it was I had going on in my head that I wasn't dealing with, I ended up throwing the shoes, my child's shoes, out of the front door.

My now frightened and tearful three-year-old child said, 'You're not angry with me. You're angry with something else, but only I am here.'

No matter how much you tell a child you love them, when you are bellowing at them, they do not feel loved. They feel the very opposite of loved. Now here I was, repeating the same behaviour I had experienced. I scooped him up, set him on the kitchen counter and held him, covering his face with kisses, endlessly telling him, 'I'm sorry, I'm sorry, Mummy is so sorry.'

I told my mum about the shoe throwing and she packed a bag and came to stay.

I also ditched the yoga and meditation classes and began Zumba classes instead.

Exercise, I discovered, helps me manage my moods immeasurably. It calms me down, lets me breathe. I got fitter and enrolled in an outdoor boot camp-type class. It was on three mornings a week. I dropped Cass at nursery and ran to the class. After a while, on the days the class was not on, my feet would be so bouncy that I put on trainers and went for long runs. I lived near Richmond Park then and could run for miles and miles in beautiful woods. This was a massive change of lifestyle for me. I could never even run for a bus before. Running was what maniacs did, but now here I was, 10km, no problem. I didn't know it then but being in nature, moving your body, are as helpful in managing ADHD as the drugs. Possibly more. But of course, a long run is not a magic fix for off-kilter brain chemistry by itself. There was still lots I had to learn.

When Cass was about ten, I was driving him to his piano lesson and we were late. It was my fault we were late. I can't remember why but I'd possibly agreed to put up a troupe of trapeze artists or decided to build an igloo just before we left the house. Being late causes me enormous anxiety. I hissed at my son, 'You weren't ready! This is YOUR fault,' while knowing full well it wasn't. But I could not stop myself. It's a vicious feeling of self-loathing when you are out of control like this. I was being unreasonable, irrational and horrible, but I couldn't do anything about it, like watching a car rolling backwards downhill without the handbrake on.

This rage came up as we hit another red light, comically late for the lesson now. 'You are SO privileged!' I roared at my son, because I had made us late for his piano lesson. 'You have no idea how bloody lucky you are and you DON'T appreciate it.' My son just sat calmly as ranted. '*I* didn't have piano lessons when I was a kid! You have everything! Do you appreciate it? NO!'

Nothing I was saying was making any sense, yet I carried on until I ran out of steam and sobbed.

My son looked over to me and smiled. 'Have you finished now?' he asked.

I nodded and took the tissue he gave me.

'Okay, Mummy. I think we should just go home,' said my boy gently.

'Okay, son.'

As we drove back, the post-tantrum exhaustion hit me and the shame scampered in. 'I'm really sorry about that, Cass,' I said. 'Listen, this is important. I don't ever want you to think that the way mummy behaved just now was normal, okay?'

Cass raised his eyebrows and said, 'Oh, don't you worry. I don't.'

Friends and family made excuses for me because they love me. 'But you are a single parent, of course you'll get stressed. You have to be kind to yourself – we ALL mess up sometimes.'

Yes, we do. All this is true. But taking my frustrations out on my children was unacceptable.

Despite loving my children with all my being, despite all the wonderful times, the gorgeous memories, the many times I got things absolutely right, I have had to face up to the fact that there were times that I failed them. Love is not enough. 'I love you' means nothing without being loving. When I shouted at my children, they didn't feel like I loved them. When you have lost your temper, you know you still love your children, you know you would still die for them, but all they see is that the person who looks after them, the person who is their world, is bigger than them, is supposed to look after them, is snarling at them. Shouting at children makes them feel hated: there is no dressing that up any other way to feel better about ourselves as parents. I have had to own it and try to fix it.

STIG OF THE DUMP

Sarah asked me quietly, 'Do you have ADHD?' Sarah was a professional declutterer and hired by the BBC to come to my house and sort out my mess for a radio show.

The production team were setting up the recording equipment while Sarah examined the gigantic piles of paperwork and boxes and boxes stuffed with photos. I expected her to be mock-horrified by the mess my paperwork was in. I thought the radio show we were making, called *Get Organised*, would mainly be her playfully tut-tutting over my ineptitude, like an admin Trinny and Susannah. I would agree, of course. 'I know! What am I like? I'm such an idiot!'

I was floored by her question. Although, she wasn't actually asking me. In a very kind, understanding and compassionate way, she was telling me. And it made sense to me. In that moment, Sarah, who I had known for approximately four-and-a-half minutes, made me understand myself more than anyone else had been able to in my whole life.

She did not treat me like an idiot. She explained that it's very common for people with ADHD to struggle to do admin – starting it seems like this impossible task, like there is a force field around it you cannot penetrate. But she was an expert at helping people like me.

Wait – there were other people like me?! Just like with bulimia, finding out that other people also have the behaviours you do – the behaviours that you have spent your life trying to hide, that have caused you shame – means that shame starts to lift. The lights in your world start to come on.

I had known I wasn't just careless. I had tried – like with homework, like with controlling my emotions – to open my post, pay my bills, keep on top of my admin, but I could not. I had hidden this mess. It had grown and suffocated me.

Admin and not being able to find things in my mess were massive triggers for my bulimia. When people knew I was bulimic they would often say, 'But you're not fat!' How could I explain, 'I know, but you see, I am throwing up my food because I have to renew my passport and I can't find my shoes.' Before I was diagnosed and started to figure out how to corral the mad horses that run through my brain, it's not that I wouldn't try to tidy: I just couldn't. Just like I couldn't perform heart surgery. I mean, I can have a bash, but it won't lead to anything good. (To be clear, I still can't do heart surgery. That is not the 'surprise turn' this book is going to take.)

I was constantly called *shelakhteh* by my gran and other family members. In Farsi, it means 'slovenly' or 'sluttish', in the original use of that word to mean 'messy'. It's a gendered insult, usually directed at women who are supposed to be ladylike and keep house, neither of which, with the best will in the world, are in my skill set.

'Ah!' my gran would tell me. 'Your cousin Lily is not like this; she is the same age as you but her bedroom is beautiful! She folds everything so beautifully.'

I hated my cousin Lily and her folded clothes.

But I couldn't be tidy. Tried. I failed. Every single time.

My house keeping style was more Stig of the Dump than Marie Kondo.

I'd fold two items of laundry then think 'washing up!' I would dump the laundry where it was and go to the sink and put on my Marigolds. As I washed a cup, I would then panic: 'Vacuum! I need to vacuum!'

And off the gloves would go and I'd get the hoover out, plug it in, then wander off to clean the loo. I would trip over the vacuum cleaner about 70 times, before finally packing it away without using it because I needed to dust first. I would sit down to do my writing then get lost in Twitter for three hours.

I couldn't understand *why* everything was still a mess, because I had been tidying for hours. Now, I make a list and cross it all off as I go. I literally write:

- Wash up
- Clear table (put things back in cupboards)
- Vacuum
- Put vacuum away
- Now
- Clean loo.

(Yes, I do have a cleaner. This is what I do before she comes over because I used to be a cleaner and I know how judge-mental *I* was.)

❁

Looking back, the signs were there in my family. Especially with my dad. Once, my brother, my mum and I went on holiday for a week without him. We got back to find my father had used every plate in the house and instead of washing up, he had gone out and bought paper plates as he still had guests round every night. He overfed the goldfish, killed them and bought two more so we wouldn't notice. They died too (my deepest apologies to the goldfish community).

My brother also, it is fair to say, is no domestic goddess. I dropped in on him unexpectedly with my daughter one afternoon. We rang the bell. He looked out from an upstairs window and wouldn't let me in. He was spooked to see us. 'Shap', he said, his eyes full of shame and panic. 'It's a mess. I can't let you see it.' I related to this.

'Have you got a dead body on your living room floor?' I shouted up. He shook his head. 'Okay, so everything is fixable.'

He opened the door. The corner sofa I had given him months earlier was still upright in the middle of his living room. The place was clean, the bathroom immaculate, but you could not see any of the floor. Clothes, books and paper – masses and masses of paper – covered every surface. My poor brother. I understood this. But – and this is interesting, I think – because it was not my own space, I could help Peyvand.

I don't know if this sounds surprising or not, but for me tidying and organising other people's space is not only not a problem, but it's actually quite a pleasure. I'm not emotionally invested in someone else's pots and pans and their other paraphernalia, so it's easy. Therapeutic. Like building Lego.

Tidying for yourself if you have ADHD is an emotionally gruel-
ling exercise. Because of the disastrous lack of focus, you end up
avoiding it. Then you leave it for so long, it gets out of hand and
feels even more insurmountable. You feel like a terrible person.
The same applies with admin. You don't open your post for
so long, you are likely to find months-old unpaid traffic fines,
uncashed cheques (my brother had post from the 2000s) and,
in my case, court summonses. Very stressful. In confronting it,
you are opening yourself up to facing how needlessly hard you
have made life for yourself and how much money you have
lost. It becomes too daunting, so you leave it and it gets worse
and worse and you feel more and more shame.

I shared a room with Peyvand until he was 13 and I was
12. Our room remained a communal space and the mess we
made was constant. Our giant bookcase was stuffed full and
nothing ever seemed to be rehomed. Andy Pandy sat side
by side with *Creative Process in Gestalt Therapy*, and Adrian
Edmonson's *How to be a Complete Bastard* with Peter and Jane.
We constantly went to the library and returned the books
three months late.

My social life has been hugely affected by my disorganisation.
I have turned up to the wrong pub, on the wrong day; I have
got so hopelessly lost and become so distressed that I have
arrived at parties in tears of frustration. 'Shappi's arrived! Get
her a drink! And a therapist!'

One New Year's Eve I invited 15 of my friends over
for a party. 'We'll eat before we come,' they all said. 'No!'

I insisted. 'I will do dinner!' Dinner for 15 people, plus ourselves, requires planning and organisation. I didn't do any of that. I woke up on New Year's Eve morning and said, 'Let's go to Richmond Park.' 'Is that a good idea?' my son asked. He seemed to be suggesting that there might be other things that needed doing, such as shopping and cooking for 15 people.

My quest to have THE PERFECT DAY overrode his concerns and off we went. We got lost after we came out of the Isabella Plantation and couldn't find our car. If you are not familiar with the size of Richmond Park, just know it took me two and a half hours to find my car. My toddler, my son and I tramped around the freezing park, with me getting more and more frantic. All I can hope is that the memory of me uselessly running around a gigantic parkland, sobbing and shrieking, 'WHICH FUCKING WAY IS IT? This park is a TOTAL CUNT' will fade in time.

By the time we got home, it was five o'clock. I hadn't been shopping or cleaned up. My guests were due at eight o'clock. I was exhausted from the two-hour tantrum I had had in the park and also filled with shame because, once again, my children had seen me behave like a two-year-old in a supermarket who was tired *and* hungry. I called my friend Lida. Lida is what I call a 'proper Iranian'. By that I mean she can conjure up banquets out of thin air. I have the Iranian sense of hospitality; I do not have the skills to back it up. When she received my SOS, she gathered things she already had in her fridge and freezer, drove over and magically laid out the most incredible Persian spread, which wowed my friends. And, yes, I allowed them to believe that I'd done everything.

I am not proud of any of this, by the way. This is just a further illustration of how I have, throughout my life, created needlessly stressful episodes because I take on too much and forget what I am capable of and what I am not.

I turned up to my wedding on the right day but left all the organising to my friend Chloe. She wasn't a wedding planner, just a friend who said, 'You can't just book the venue, you have to sort out food, music, all that stuff. It's in September! It's already August, you haven't got much time!'

'Sure!' I said. 'I know all that!' And off I went to the Edinburgh Festival, hoping that Chloe would do it all. And she did. Chloe and my mother did everything.

The one job I had was to send out the invitations. I got some of the evening and ceremony ones muddled up so some of my dearest friends were hurt they'd only been invited to the evening do and some people I hardly knew sat and watched us exchange our vows. If I hadn't shirked my responsibilities, the wedding dinner would have been Doritos and dips and everyone would have danced to my dad playing the spoons. It is always in the interest of everyone if I have nothing to do with organising anything.

If ADHD means my interactions with people are chaotic, it is similarly merciless when it comes to my dealings with the inanimate objects in my life. I have spent a significant amount of my time on this planet looking for things that were 'in my hand a second ago!' I have, at one point or another, been unable to find most of my possessions when I need them. Many times, I have thought that if burglars broke into my house, they would think someone had beaten them to it.

For years, I have toured as a stand-up and yet I have never, ever learned the skills I need to leave the house in any kind of ordered, calm way. It has always been a flurry of 'I'm late for my train!' as I dash around stuffing essentials in my suitcase at the last minute, turning the house upside down looking for my phone or purse.

I plan much better now that I know how to calm my brain down. I am easier on myself but it's been the part of having ADHD that has made people think it's HILARIOUS to take the piss out of. The type who see you climb through the window of your own house once and after that, every time they see you snigger, 'Hoo hoo hoo, you haven't locked yourself out again, have you?' No. I am in the Co-op buying lemons.

The sheer rudeness of some people when you are not immediately efficient IS unbelievable. People have watched me and laughed as I scrambled around frantically in my bag for my phone or keys, or stood by and smirked as I struggled with filling in a form or the self-checkout machine. Just because I once promised I'd pick up a neighbour's child from school, forgot and got a call from the school as I was boarding a plane to Sweden, there are some people who still will say 'You definitely can pick up my girls? Are you sure? I'm not going to call you and find you are in Hawaii? Hahaha!' I would like to see any of these people grappling with a neurological condition they don't know they have *and* be able to remember they're supposed to be in Thailand in the morning. When I didn't know I had ADHD, I'd flush with shame when I made mistakes. But now, I dare anyone to call me 'Scatty Shappi' or take the piss.

Finally, in my forties, I began to stand up to people who mocked my mistakes at a charity quiz I was hosting (Yes, my moment of standing up to bullies finally came at a sweet charity event and not a karaoke tournament with Mr Miagi by my side, sadly). The teams were made up of the heads of major TV companies, television commissioners and heads of huge tech companies, and I unravelled. I had never hosted a quiz before and fumbled the questions. At one point, one of the organisers had to go up and repeat a question I had garbled. In the break, I passed one of the tables and a man on it hissed, 'You literally just had to read some instructions in order' in front of all of the other people at his table. I could feel that familiar shame of being laughed at because I was not able to do something which seemed simple to others.

I tried to style it out: 'I was a *bit* unclear, but I *think* I got away with it.' He was set on humiliating me, though, and as his companions looked on, he said, 'No. You didn't. *Who* booked *you?*' So many times in a situation like this, tears have sprung. But here I was, on my one night off in a fortnight and instead of being at home with my children, I had agreed to this charity gig, which I wasn't being paid for, and now someone was being horrible to me. I met his contemptuous stare with quite a contemptuous one of my own, said 'Fuck off' and walked away. It felt good. I really don't know why it took me so long.

Knowing that I have ADHD and understanding more about how my brain is wired does not, of course, mean I am 'cured'. I still get muddled, struggle with organisation and time keeping, but I now have the confidence to say to people, 'I am sorry. I did reply to your urgent email. I replied in my head, but realise you would not have seen that. I hope you found the help you needed and are no longer in a prison in Turkey.'

I have arrived in the wrong cities, on the wrong days. I have turned up at meetings and not realised I was supposed to have a pitch prepared. When I turned up to a wedding a week early, the couple in question, friends of my parents, were very sweet and invited me in. They had a huge, fancy home which was being prepared for the extravaganza the following week. The couple were in their pyjamas and insisted I stay for pancakes; I was in a full wedding guest outfit, complete with present. I once had a gig at the Leicester Square Theatre on a Saturday night and, 20 minutes before the show, not a single person had turned up to be in my audience. I was gutted. This was it. The end of my career.

I steeled myself and asked the lad at the box office: 'How many tickets were sold?'

He tappy-tip-tapped on his computer and said, 'Six!' as encouragingly as he could. It was a 400-seater theatre.

I said, 'How would it be if I cancelled?'

He lit up. 'Oh, that would mean I could get an earlier train to Birmingham to see my girlfriend!'

Go, I told him. Go and be young and happy and in love while I cry in the rain, wondering how I will feed and clothe my children. I called my brother and sobbed. He reassured me that *he* would feed and clothe us if it came to it, and told me to join him for a drink. I jumped in a rickshaw. Whigfield's 'Saturday Night' blared from its speakers, drowning out my crying. My brother and his friends had bought me a vat of wine which I gratefully guzzled down. My phone rang; it was my agent.

'I cancelled!' I told him, already tipsy. 'There were only six tickets sold and I couldn't bear it.'

My agent, who had known me for some time now, gently but urgently asked, 'Which theatre did you go to?'

'The Leicester Square Theatre,' I replied

'Right. Three hundred people are waiting for you at The Arts Theatre, Covent Garden. I'll tell them you're on your way.'

The joy and relief as I flew there was incredible. I started a little late but I explained what had happened and had enormous fun. To this day, I do not know whose show I waltzed into the Leicester Square Theatre and cancelled.

I once got a county court judgement against me because I hadn't opened my post. And when I was so skint that I used to often eat Weetabix and banana for my dinner, I failed to cash a cheque for £50. I couldn't get it together to take it to the bank. It seems easy enough, doesn't it? Grab your paperwork, put on some clothes, matching shoes, get your phone, keys and wallet and leave the house. Go and sort your shit out at the bank. But I would spend whole days in my bedsit trying to do this and still could not. I would pick up the paperwork, forget where I put it (in a bedsit, may I remind you) then I'd find some shoes, maybe I'd suddenly decide I needed a bath and then perhaps I would have some toast but end up eating eight slices instead of two, then I would make myself sick and get into the bulimia fog. Hours could go by like this, then maybe days. The next thing you know, you are packing to leave the bedsit a year later and you find an out-of-date cheque for £50.

I thought life would be easier when I got internet banking but I frequently forget passwords. I get locked out and cry on the phone to my bank, who tell me, 'Click on the link, take three strands of a mermaid's hair, shavings from a unicorn's horn, sacrifice a small trout and once you've scanned all that to us, we will send you a white dove who will reset your password, in return for your daughter's hand in marriage.' This is what I hear anyway.

My ADHD is avoidant of anything to do with finance. It's a fear of facing what could be years of being underpaid. I posted on Twitter about how much I was not able to deal with organising my paperwork. This was what led Amy Wheel, a producer at BBC Radio 4, to get in touch and set me up with Sarah the declutterer. Amy had been commissioned to make a show about the fad of decluttering and thought I would be a good person to feature in it. She wanted to get me to do some decluttering tasks and record my progress. (Later,

I put up a post about how much I longed to travel first class to Bermuda and stay for a month at a five-star beach resort, all expenses paid. Nothing as yet from the BBC on *that*.)

I was suspicious of Sarah when she arrived at my house. She was an attractive, very soft-voiced Australian with huge blue eyes. Was she going to judge me? Was she going to tut, tell me the errors of my ways before rolling all my socks into tiny balls and throwing away my favourite dresses?

What she actually did was to go through my gigantic pile of paperwork, which was almost as tall as me (5 foot 2 inches so not all that bad) and reduce it to seven smart folders, beautifully ordered, with everything clearly marked so keeping them organised was easy.

Making the radio programme was cathartic and unexpectedly emotional. I wasn't expecting to blub while showing Sarah my piles of boxes of photos. Living with us was the family's archive of pictures dating back to the early 1900s. They filled a whole wardrobe. As a child, I spent hours looking through them all, swearing that one day I would sort them out, rescue them from the precarious life they had, all bundled into trunks and book boxes. When Sarah got to them, there were pictures of me drunk at a party in my student days mixed up with photos of my mum as a toddler, along with a whole roll of pictures of a school trip which seemed to be mostly of the wheels of the coach. The photos had, over the years, become an impossible-to-climb mountain, getting bigger and bigger. They weighed me down. Even though I had stuffed them in a cupboard and closed the door, I felt their presence: I knew that if I didn't sort them out, one day I would be gone and my children, in their grief, would wonder if they should keep the photo of their mother aged 19, at an Ann Summers party, sucking on a dildo.

In the radio programme (you can still find it online), you can clearly hear me become teary when Sarah pulls out some photos of my son's third birthday. I had not looked at them since I had them developed almost ten years earlier. They represented a sealed box of shut away, unprocessed, painful emotions I hadn't wanted to face. Cass's third birthday was the first he had after his dad and I split, the first when he didn't have his mum *and* dad with him. Christian and I were not getting along, and he was having a separate party with our son the next day.

I was desperately sad. I could not put it into perspective. I had failed my boy and that was that. He was too young to understand all this grotty adult stuff. *I* couldn't understand it and I *was the* grotty adult. This sadness, these rows between Christian and I had no business in the life of this happy child who greeted every morning by singing out to me from his bed: 'Mummy! It's a lovely da-ay!'

I'd pulled out all the stops. All his little buddies crammed into our kitchen: everyone was a pirate, my friend made a glorious cake and I focused on him having the best, most lovely day possible. But now, ten years on, when I looked at the photos – saw myself looking so young, holding my boy to me, smiling for the camera but my glassy eyes frantic with pain – I was right back there, in the kitchen of our old house, when I was wild with heartache. This was the danger these photographs held for me – the reason I'd been scared to tackle them. We had moved on since then: Christian lived nearby, we got on, his partner was a loving part of our lives. But opening that box had exposed raw grief still howling and beating as I had got on with my life.

Later that day, after we finished recording, my children and I went for a pizza and my son texted his dad to join us. Christian popped in and shared a pizza with us. This man sitting with us in a pizzeria that day, sharing our food, laughing with the kids was nothing to do with the feelings I'd had earlier. He brought up none of the feelings the photos did. I was completely at ease with *this* guy. All the emotions had been locked away with the clutter of my photos. No wonder they had been impossible to sort out all these years.

Sarah helped me conquer them, and all the grief, joy and sentiment they guarded. We went through my boxes of photos together at first until she recognised key family members and friends, then I left her to it. She threw hundreds away (always giving me a glance at them first), deciding I didn't need seven pictures of a chicken I took on a school trip in 1983, or ones of just half of someone's face, or pictures of complete strangers at parties I do not remember attending. By looking at the fashions and the paper they were printed on, Sarah was able to magically put them in chronological order. Now they are in seven smart, labelled, waterproof, shoebox-sized boxes *and* on a hard drive. I can pick an event or a year and find the pictures from that time in a moment.

Facing my photo clutter was an emotional purge. Our clutter is a reflection of how we manage our emotions, what we hold on to, what we cannot let go. Decluttering is not about being house-proud, it's about being present in your own life as it is today. I didn't throw away the photos of my son's third birthday, of course, but I finally acknowledged the grief they held for that period in my life. I can look at them now with fondness rather than agony.

My ADHD brain locked me away in daydreams to avoid confronting feelings. Bulimia and other compulsive behaviours I had were a part of that sealing away of feelings. If you have ADHD you might relate to how elusive a feeling can be as you lock yourself away. You 'check out' of yourself. You try to escape yourself. But nothing goes away; all the unresolved stuff in your life – your grief, your anger, your pain, your fucking admin – grows and grows and engulfs you until you are in a fog and unable to manage this precious bit of life you have been given and live it in a way that brings you peace.

A formal ADHD diagnosis was still a few years off, but talking to Sarah, understanding this was quite likely a pathological issue, was freedom. I cannot do admin just as I cannot do a triple backflip. I will not spend time trying to do a triple backflip.

I asked Sarah to help my dad with his hoarding and clutter. I showed her pictures of his office and his garage. She looked at the pictures – my dad's piles and piles of papers and books and puppets he had made. Relics of mine and Peyvand's child-hood he had kept. Every inch of the walls was covered with pictures; the floor was crowded with furniture he insisted was 'antique', musical instruments he doesn't play and, inexplicably, a traffic cone. Possessions and objects he insists have sentimental value and would never let me sort.

Sarah looked at them all then asked, simply, 'Did he suffer a loss in early childhood?'

Wow. She was spot on. 'Well', I told her, 'his dad died when he was six and he was sent to live in the city, away from his mum.'

'I can't help,' she said, gently. 'This clutter doesn't bother him. It might bother you and your mum, but he needs this. People, especially of your dad's generation, who lost a parent at a time when children's mental health wasn't considered, often cannot throw anything away. It's all tied in with loss.'

I thought of this again when I read Billy Connolly's autobiography, where he describes the room he writes and plays music in. He writes about it in all its cluttered, bric-a-brac glory with stuff everywhere. He says that homes that are very ordered, well-designed and organised are 'too rehearsed'. His mum left him when he was four and the other adults in his life were brutal to him. His room sounded similar to my dad's.

When Sarah moved back to Australia after the pandemic, I was bereft. Her soothing voice and her intricate knowledge of shredders had become integral to the smooth running of my life. She will forever be a part of my life in the form of the still-exquisitely organised admin binders she got for me (I also have her email address).

Clare was one of the mums from my daughter's year who reminded me of the girls at my own school, the ones who always looked smart, knew exactly what we were meant to be doing in class and never had anything weird like rice or kebabs in their packed lunch. 'Your house is so *clutter free!*' I said when I went to her home for the first time. I told her about Sarah and how she had changed my life by decluttering my photos and my admin and how sad I was that she had moved to the other side of the world. While she had sorted out the really emotionally debilitating things, my house remained messy, with shoes, books and bric-a-brac everywhere. I told Clare about how I had begun to think I had ADHD and how I could not keep up with myself when it came to putting things away.

Clare said, 'Decluttering is my passion. Do you want me to help you?'

I looked at her, this woman whose home was perfect, and said solemnly, 'Help me, Clare from the School Run. You're my only hope.'

Clare came over and got stuck in like a builder, demolishing and building back up again. With firm compassion, she helped put about two-thirds of my belongings in the charity shop. Clare gently explained that I did not need three can openers and reduced the pots, pans, dishes and utensils in my kitchen down to just what I need. I had beautiful dishes and vases which were swamped in the backs of cupboards. She brought out the lovely things and displayed them. 'Use them. Every day is a special occasion. Nothing is "for best". Don't hide away your pretty things.'

That afternoon, I picked my daughter up from school in a ball-gown. Clare had stripped my wardrobe down to just the clothes I loved or the ones that were practical necessities. According to Clare, 67 pairs of knickers was excessive, so we whittled them down to 25. I had to debate quite robustly with her about activewear but, in the end, had to concede that 17 pairs of Lycra leggings, some dating back to 1999, was too much. We just kept the 3 that fit best. I could feel myself coming round to the idea that I did not need to keep clothes that didn't fit me just in case I grew or shrunk. I was not, Clare reminded me, Alice in Wonderland.

As our rapport grew, Clare became more honest. 'This has had its day, hasn't it?' she said, and tossed the tacky camisole I had had for 15 years in the 'to go' pile. I told Clare I am always losing things. She said, 'Do you ever lose your toothbrush?'

Point made. Of course I never lose my toothbrush. It is always, *always,* in the dog basket.

WHY I ACTUALLY THREW THE CADBURY MILK TRAY

I was walking to my friend's house, during the first Covid-19 lockdown. Breathing was tricky due to the sobbing and I was halfway down the road before I realised I was just in my socks. I ploughed on. This was an emergency. I had just destroyed a box of Cadbury Milk Tray, in the midst of a global pandemic.

Anxiety was fierce at that point for many of us. Thousands were dying around the world and we felt like we might die too if someone blinked vigorously within 6 feet of us. All my work disappeared and we didn't know at the start how Covid would affect children. How did I know I wasn't going to die from it? My mum and dad both had severe health problems. Would I lose them? How was I going to pay for my house now that my industry had disappeared? Fortunately, at least there were not many people around to see me sobbing and snotting my way through the high street.

Up until this day, I had been good at hiding my fears about Covid from my children. I did not put on the news. Every morning when I went into the kitchen, I smashed on *The Chris Evans Breakfast Show*. His relentless, unbending positivity and happy music was what I needed. The children did not always want to come on early morning dog walks, which was a blessing as it gave me space to have panic attacks privately, in bushes, minimising the risk of me screaming, 'WE ARE ALL GOING TO DIE' at breakfast.

It was a time when we found out how many regard our basic human needs as food, shelter, water and … bog roll. Every time I left home to go to buy food, I felt like I was risking all our lives. In those early weeks of the first lockdown, we were all little shipwrecked units, trying to survive. There was so little we knew for sure about the virus that no one seemed to know which way was up and which was down.

A few weeks into lockdown one, I was scouring the near-empty supermarket shelves, finding obscure brand canned meat and assuring myself that the war generation lived on this stuff and all survived to be 103. I saw a flash of purple right at the back of one of the higher shelves … a box of Cadbury Milk Tray! What a find! I stood on my tiptoes, stretched my arm across the shelf and teased it to me with my fingertips, delighted and proud that I, the lioness, would be taking my cubs such a comforting and familiar treat in these unfamiliar times.

I flung myself back into my house, triumphant. 'Look what I've got!' I said, and gave the chocolates to my children. I beamed as they tried to open the box. I was a successful hunter-gatherer. I could do this. I could keep my ship sailing through the storm.

My children, being children, squabbled when opening the box. 'It's this way!' and 'Gimme it, I know how to do it!' This minor, very ordinary bit of sibling kerfuffle flicked a switch and my facade of calm was blown clean away.

Suddenly, I was pure fury. I grabbed the box and ripped it open, sending chocolates scattering up in the air and all over the floor. Our two dogs leapt up and flew to scavenge treats. My children, knowing chocolate is dangerous for dogs, also flew at the chocolates. I stood shrieking at the top of my voice, something along the lines of, 'I have had enough! YOU HAVE NO IDEA HOW FUCKING LUCKY YOU ARE! YOU CHOCOLATES! WE ARE JUST A PANDEMIC HOW DARE YOU? I DIDN'T HAVE PIANO LESSONS WHEN I WAS A KID!' I was not making a great deal of sense.

My children calmed the dogs and Cass put the now-tainted chocolates in the bin. The look he gave me from his giant, soulful eyes said, 'That was not okay.'

I had lost control. This was not fair. I needed help. Apart from feeding and clothing them, I was also responsible for not screaming my lungs out at them when they opened a box of chocolates from the wrong end. So I left the house in my socks and called my neighbour, who has keys to my house.

'I have gone mad. Can you keep an eye on my kids?'

She instantly understood and reassured me that she would. 'I'll go and sit in your front garden,' she said. After I left she texted me: 'Breathe. You are not alone.'

I know, I thought. *The whole street must have heard me.*

I sat in my friend's garden, rocking backwards and forwards for a good while. I had known this friend since childhood and mumbled, slightly wild-eyed, about what had happened. She well-meaningly said, 'Well, I imagine children CAN be annoying, especially if you are cooped up all day with them.'

She lent me some shoes to go home in and I left. *She was wrong*, I thought. My children had not been annoying. I had been the annoying, irrational one. They were not the problem. Children are never the problem. I loved being cooped up with them. Our normal lives revolved around goodbyes because I travelled constantly for my work. 'I wish I could be home ALL the time,' I frequently wailed to my family.

In lockdown, I absolutely loved being home to cook for them every day and going to bed snuggled up with my youngest. I was making up for lost time. It was delicious. My children had not driven me to 'lose it' anymore than I drove my dad to 'lose it' when I was a child. This cycle needed to be broken.

I had a responsibility to get to the bottom of why I had these over-the-top reactions to minor irritations. In normal times, our lives and home were full of family, friends and neighbours. When I was a tetchy and shouty mum when I was stressed out, which was often, there was usually someone else around to lend a hand so I calmed down quickly and apologised. Or I took my stress outside of the house. Now, my children were alone with me indefinitely: I was all they had. They were cooped up with *me*. They needed me to not lose my shit and hurl good chocolate about the place. They needed to have a home they felt safe in, not one where they trod on eggshells around their mother. Enough of blaming my childhood, bulimia, bullies at school, my divorce, the government, a shitty personality … all of these things might play a part, but something else was locking me in to this behaviour cycle. Why was I behaving in ways that were contrary to my values?

'Right, kids', I said to my children. My six-year-old daughter clung to me and my big boy made me a cup of tea. Thank goodness for talk about mental health in schools these days. Thank goodness that at the ages of 6 and 12, my children were able to take it on board when I said, 'My mental health is not good at the moment. You did nothing wrong. Absolutely nothing. I am sorry. I am going to get some help from a special kind of doctor who helps with mental health.' Then we baked a cake and watched *Brooklyn Nine-Nine*.

I typed *Therapist ADHD London* into the search box on my computer.

Up flashed centres and kind-looking therapists who specialised in adult ADHD; teen ADHD; childhood ADHD. I remembered the bulimia therapist I had seen three times, who I caught watching the clock, who kept trying to make me do a food plan then stood me up. I was older now, confident about getting help, and I wanted a proper, spill-your-guts, tell-me-things-you-wouldn't-even-write-in-your-diary therapist.

On the website for the British Association for Counselling and Psychotherapy (UKCP), I found Ian. He was a psychoanalytic psychotherapist. The two 'psychos' in his job title were reassuring. I liked that his emails were professional without being cold, spelling out his terms and conditions, letting me know that the first session was just to see if we wanted to see if we might want to work together; that there was no obligation to have a second. This was a relief. I just wouldn't get in touch again if I didn't connect with him, rather than fake my own death to avoid the awkwardness of saying, 'I don't want to make another appointment.' (This is standard in therapy, by the by, I discovered. You should never be asked to commit to sessions straight away.)

On his UKCP page it listed ADHD as one of the things he could help with. I trusted him immediately.

'I'm not here to "fix" you or give you advice,' he told me. 'I am here to support you.' Support is a very different thing to advice. I had had enough of advice. 'What you need to do … if you would just …' was useless, but there is only so much your friends and family and taxi drivers can do to help you. (There are taxi drivers all over the UK who have heard the A–Z of my divorce in the days when it was literally all I could talk about. Thank you, if you happen to read this, Thomas, Mohammed, Majcek, Pete from Norwich and all the others who were so patient and kind with their over-sharing passenger.)

Quite early on, while I was talking about my marriage breaking up, Ian looked at me with such empathy that it hurt, in a way that was a release, a validation of what I had been through. Some painful emotions around certain periods of my life were still boxed up, fully intact. They sat inside me like raging fires. *Best not look.* But nothing healed by me ignoring it. They gnawed away at me and spilled out in ways that damaged me and hurt the people I loved (and occasionally people I did not love, like the rude guy on a bus who suddenly found himself being shrieked at by a woman with a baby in a papoose, brandishing a mop she had just bought).

Therapy helped me understand and unpick my thought processes. It was like untangling a 10-foot string of fairy lights after it had been put away on Christmas Day by a knot enthusiast. Talking to Ian is how I imagine my dog felt when I finally got a professional dog trainer. 'You see? I'm not mad! This person understands me! This person speaks my language.'

The more we untangled, the more I processed emotions I had shut in a drawer and left waiting. Ian and I had sessions three times a week for the first few months. On Zoom, of course, as we were in lockdown. This is a lot of money at the best of times, even more so as I wasn't earning, but I would have sold my possessions if I'd had to. What Ian was doing for me was priceless. There was a huge backlog we needed to get through and even though I was often a sobbing bag of snot after a session, I knew that this was the beginning of a meaningful change for the better in how I lived my life. I could feel myself healing, physically healing. My whole body felt lighter.

ADHD is not curable: just manageable. In the middle of one session, I had been talking for some time, lying on my sofa and propping the computer on the arm, when Ian said gently, 'Now, Shappi, I need to disclose something to you.'

Oh my God! What was he going to say? Was he in love with me? I knew he was engaged, and to a man. This was huge!

'As you know, I have ADHD.' Yes, I knew that. He had told me in our first session.

'As you were speaking,' he very earnestly continued, 'I picked up my phone and I answered a WhatsApp message from you.'

Oh, I thought. As I often forgot the times and days of our sessions, I'd texted Ian just before to confirm our session was at 2pm today. Seeing my message, he'd responded 'yes', at 2.08pm. WHILE WE WERE HAVING OUR SESSION. Pure ADHD.

'Right,' I said.

'Yes', said Ian. 'So when you finish this session and turn your phone back on, you'll find a message from me, answering your WhatsApp message, and it will have been sent in the middle of our session.'

'Right,' I said again.

'Can you take a moment and try to tell me how you feel about your therapist absent-mindedly messaging you in the middle of a session?'

'I think,' I told him, 'that is absolutely hilarious.' And I did. I laughed until I was crying. 'Please, Ian, please tell me you've been playing Candy Crush all throughout our sessions?'

He allowed himself a smile. 'I have not.'

He sat patiently until I stopped hysterically laughing, which took a while. Eventually I wiped my eyes and said, 'I think it's brilliant. I think it's brilliant you didn't even make the connection that it was me you were texting. That's champion ADHD-ing!'

The conversation about how it made me feel was important, he told me. I examined whether it was the people-pleasing part of me, trying to be a 'good' client. But no, I was sure it was because I found it genuinely funny and very relatable.

Ian's manner, intelligence and way of working suited me; he was kind, compassionate, honest and I felt at home.

❄

After a few months of therapy, Ian asked me how I would feel about taking medication. He explained a little about the different types, but told me an experienced psychiatrist would have to complete an ADHD assessment first and, if appropriate, give me a prescription. I booked to speak to a psychiatrist a friend recommended.

The waiting lists for diagnosis are horribly long. I was able to pay to go privately, but if you can't do this, there are brilliant online resources that can help you while you wait for official diagnosis. Official diagnosis means you can get the medication but, as I have mentioned before, medication is just one of the ways you can manage ADHD.

A friend I met on dog walks told me about *ADDitude* magazine. Reading big textbooks is hard for my jumping jack brain, but this website is clear and so helpful. I watched TEDx Talks given by people with ADHD. Salif Mahamane's was the first one I watched. I had never heard anyone speak so eloquently about these challenges that I had had all my life but did not know how to articulate, that I tried to keep hidden. Absorbing information, hearing other people's experiences, was exhilarating! These people understood; they shared my experience. I learned about my own behaviour patterns and what was down to deficiency in my neurotransmitters. For me, ADHD was not a disability, it did not mean there was anything wrong with me: it was just a different set up.

No wonder so many self-employed people have ADHD, I thought, *when other people's rules can be impossible to understand and follow.* A study conducted by The ADHD Foundation in 2022 found that a high percentage of people in prison have ADHD too. They are now campaigning to have ADHD screening in prisons to help people understand it and lower the risk of repeat offending.

I had already started to find out more about how to manage my mental health before I started to address my issues more directly with Ian and learn about ADHD. But I was in my forties by the time it had become normal for people to talk about their mental health and, at the same time, there was a conversation around neurodivergence. But for my whole life, I had been told that the things I struggled with were my own fault – I wasn't focusing enough, I wasn't working hard enough, I didn't care enough. I was labelled 'a dipstick', 'mental', 'aggressive', 'lazy'. 'Scatty Shappi'. My internal monologue repeated these things to me, caused me to ruminate endlessly on negative thoughts and feelings, making anxiety feel immovable, a permanent fixture inside me.

I broke the cycle of dating men who belittled or controlled me. I had got myself to a place, by running and reading and listening to heaps of mental health podcasts, where I understood and felt that being single and content was a gift. I love Viv Albertine's book *Clothes, Clothes, Clothes. Music, Music, Music. Boys, Boys, Boys.* and her line 'being single is like being wealthy' really stuck with me and helped me break my pattern of feeling needy if I didn't have the attention of a man.

When people ask me, 'When did you get your diagnosis?', it's not as easy to answer as just telling them the date of my appointment with the psychiatrist. The progress towards a diagnosis, understanding that my chaos and struggles were not just learned behaviour or emotional malaise took years. Our culture has shifted the taboo of talking about neuro-divergence and normalised the language around it. Young people seem to be much more clued up about mental health than I had been at that age. I consumed social media posts, watched their TEDx Talks and thought, *This is me.*

When the psychiatrist confirmed my diagnosis it was no surprise, but I cried anyway, with relief. It gave me an official answer.

My psychiatrist explained how the drug he was prescribing worked. 'It wakes up the sleepy part of your brain that organises the rest of your brain.' It was an amphetamine. That explained why I had loved whizz so much when I was younger. Most people take amphetamine recreationally to dance all night, to get high. But for many people with ADHD, your energy levels can be bonkers: you can't sleep, your focus is already bouncing because you have a deficiency which means you are not fully in control of your executive functions. The amphetamine shakes it into action.

I lost my compulsion to overeat. That is without doubt the most awesome thing the drugs did for me. I know when I have forgotten to take it because I move around the house stuffing whatever I can find into my mouth (further proof of my assertion that all dogs have ADHD). All those years I was locked in bulimia, in that ghastly addiction, unable to understand this physical urge, the unstoppable drive to eat. And now it has gone.

If I don't manage my ADHD properly and relapse with bulimia (which can happen from time to time) I am not filled with shame and self-hate; I don't feel I have undone my recovery. It feels like I have fallen over; that it was an accident and I should try to be more careful.

I maintain that for me, the drugs are nothing without therapy and nature. Running, walking the dogs, learning to say 'no' to work and social engagements which overload my plate are just as important. I hardly drink alcohol anymore because life is sweet without it. It costs me my sleep and it doesn't do well with ADHD medication. Sleep is an absolute priority. Resting is an activity, not just something that may or may not happen when you are exhausted.

My grandmothers, the older generation of my eastern culture, understood this without naming it. 'Go and have a rest' or 'I'm going to have a rest' were sentences they said a lot that never occurred to me to say. Being 'busy' does not mean you are fulfilled.

I don't look back on my school days and life before my diagnosis as a 'mess' anymore. I used to easily say, 'I was really bad at school' or 'I was crap at comedy for ages' or 'I had awful boyfriends'. But actually, I was doing brilliantly considering the things I was quietly, unknowingly dealing with. I may have gone around the houses and, as my friend Noreen put it, 'lived the lives of seven people all at once' but, in my own way, I weaved a path which finally got me to the peaceful life I have now.

Both my children notice how different I am since I began therapy. 'You never shout anymore,' they have said more than once. And, unless I have stubbed my toe, I really don't. Not at anyone. Not even angry motorists who *HONK HONK HONK!* behind the bin truck. I now go up to them and gently ask, 'Have you considered you may have ADHD?' (Relax. I don't really. Though I do think it.)

There is nothing 'wrong' with me and there never was. I am a misfit, but so are many others. Medicalising everyone who does not flow successfully through our education system and the work culture we have created is not the answer. I do not believe I have a disorder. I just don't open my post and am unlikely to remember your name. I will, however, remember every detail you tell me about your life. I will remember how many cats or dogs or children you have. I'll remember what your job is and whether you like it or not. I will constantly mull over the things we talked about. I have a vast attention span, but it may be focused entirely on looking up different species of ape when I'm in a Zoom meeting.

The therapy, the medication, the running, the occasional hugging of a tree, all help settle my mind and organise my ADHD. I meditate, too – it turns out it clears space to sort my head out and make clear decisions. Who knew?

My children may no longer have a shouty mum, but they do have a mum who misses ferries and cannot sit still for very long. I still have to pinch my palm sometimes to stop myself interrupting when someone else is talking. I am still a scatter brain, but I am able to manage my life so my scattered brain does not exhaust itself, and nor, most importantly, does it beat itself up.

We are only scratching the surface of how common ADHD is. So many of us do not have linear thinking. I struggle with all the things I have mentioned in this book, but if you need to stall a bailiff at your door while you lock away your valuables, I'm your gal. If you need someone to make a speech she knows next to nothing about, I can help. I am the friend or neighbour or colleague you will never be imposing on because I can change plans and accommodate the new with a split second's notice.

I am the person who will say 'leap and the ground will find you!' when all your other friends are telling you to be sensible. I will hold your hand and jump with you. I will take risks and scrap the 'pros and cons' list, running headlong into whatever has grabbed my attention.

The world of stand-up comedy has been a home for misfits like me. It was my escape from intolerable routine. The unrelenting energy my ADHD gave me yanked me up and made me run whenever I felt drained or helpless throughout my life.

This fizzing, rampant brain of mine is who I am. It's not a 'condition' to be fixed. Knowing about it has helped give me a break and encouraged me to stop trying to change.

Despite the mayhem I often found myself in, I have two magical children of my own, did well enough to support them both (and two dogs and two cats) and still have an exciting life. I bore the emotional avalanches of divorce and single-parenthood, alongside an intense career without understanding that my ADHD made things ten times harder than they needed to be. But, in this tiny snippet of life we have all been gifted, why dwell on the times when you had to sleep in a shed because you lost both sets of keys?

It will take a long while still to make sure work and educational spaces accommodate those of us who are not neurotypical. But, in the meantime, I take comfort in my very tidy sock drawer, where bank statements no longer lurk.

ACKNOWLEDGEMENTS

My love and thanks to my agent Cathryn Summerhayes, who is also Wonder Woman. Thanks to everyone in my Curtis Brown family, who are all kind and clever badasses. Thanks to the brilliant Sam Jackson at Penguin, who waded through the initial streams of consciousness I was trying to pass off as a book. She is Yoda-like in her patience, even though she would have been well within her rights, at least thirty-seven times, to scream 'DO YOU EVEN DEADLINE BRO?' in our Zoom meetings. Thank you to Liz Marvin for her smart slapping into shape of my 'chapters'/mountains of thoughts and stories in no particular order. Thank you also to Evangeline Stanford and to the copyeditor, Leona Skene, and proofreader, Claudia Connal, for your questions, ideas and attention to detail.

One of the most wonderful things to happen to me in the last couple of years is meeting the brain of Delyth Jones. Delyth's humour, intelligence and honesty were invaluable to me in the hours and hours we spent talking about this book. Thank you for your notes, steers and abundant humour, and for being the clever friend I needed when writing this. You are a literary wizard.

Thank you to Charlotte Wolf from across my fence, who heeded my SOS on Dairy Milk Day, and to all the people in this book who supported me when life was chaotic and I was upside down.

Thank you to Lianne and everyone at Impatient Productions for your understanding and support. Thanks also to Hollie Ebdon at Ebdon Management, everyone at Speaking Office for being completely amazing and keeping me sailing, and to Rozzy Wyatt for being my organised friend.

Thanks to Vissey and Chloe who are always there to hear my BLAH!

Thanks to all of my friends in my wonderful West London community who, whether they realised it or not, were an incredible support to me with their tea and sympathy, wine, dog walks, childcare and karaoke, especially my amazing Hali-over-the-road and Sophie, the Queen of our street. Thank you to my darling Noreen, Josephina, Lisa-from-uni-who-is-now-down-the-road, Catherine, Rachel and all your beautiful, vibrant children, who make moving back to Ealing the best decision I ever made. Thanks to Khalid and Poonam whose candid chats during dog walks gave me so much confidence to start talking publicly about ADHD.

My sincere gratitude to Ian King-Brown for your expertise and compassion, and for opening the world of psychotherapy to me.

Thank you to Heather and Andy on the Isle of Wight, for being the best neighbours when I go to write there. And also to Will, who holds the fort, takes care of my children and makes the most amazing soup when I am working.

Also, thank you to Esther Manito, brilliant stand-up comedian and superb friend, who took her sweet time coming into my life. (Being ten years younger than me is no excuse. I love you.)

I am so grateful to everyone who messaged me on social media to share your own stories and who sought me out after gigs to chat about ADHD. Talking about it was a game changer.

Thanks to my family: Nadia and Daniel for lighting up our lives, and to my mum, dad and brother Peyvand for graciously allowing me to include more painful parts of our lives and for putting up with me endlessly insisting 'WE ALL HAVE ADHD!'

This book is dedicated to my mum, who praised me and cuddled me as a child, which was so important. She is the best.

Lastly, and always mostly, thank you to my children. Cass and Vivie, it is an utter privilege to be your mum. It wasn't always easy for you before I got help for ADHD. Thank you both for being so understanding and kind. You are the funniest, smartest people I have ever met. Thank you for making my life such a fun adventure and for teaching me everything. Thank goodness for you two.

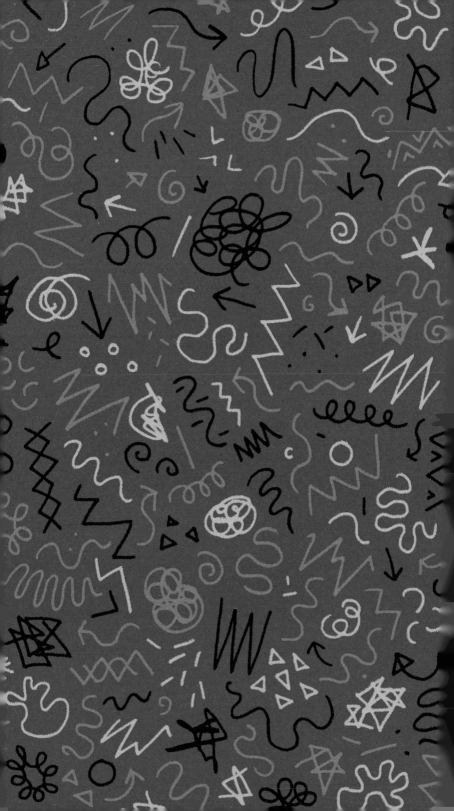